Groupwork for Children with Autism Spectrum Disorder

Ages 11–16

Groupwork for Children with Autism Spectrum Disorder

Ages 11-16

AN INTEGRATED APPROACH

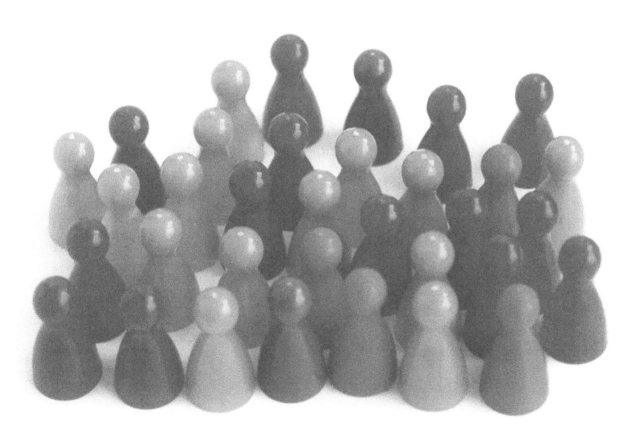

Alyson Eggett, Kerrie Old,
Liz Ann Davidson & Christina Howe

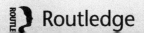
Routledge

Notes on the text

Purely for clarity, we have used the term 'he' to refer to the group member and 'she' to refer to the parent, carer or professional throughout the book.

Autism Spectrum Disorder is abbreviated to ASD throughout the text.

All the names in the book have been changed to protect the identity of the young people involved.

First published 2008 by Speechmark Publishing Ltd

Published 2017 by Routledge
2 Park Square, Milton Park, Abingdon, Oxon OX14 4RN
711 Third Avenue, New York, NY 10017, USA

Routledge is an imprint of the Taylor & Francis Group, an informa business

British Library Cataloguing in Publication Data

Groupwork for children with autism spectrum disorder : an integrated approach
  Ages 11–16
    1. Autistic children – Education 2. Group work in education
    I. Eggett, Alyson
    371.9'4395

ISBN: 9780863885952 (pbk)

Contents

List of activities

WARM-UP/ROUND-UP GAMES

1   Parachute games

LEARNING ABOUT OURSELVES

2   People bingo
3   Interviews
4   Show and tell
5   Feely bags
6   Friendship darts
7   Compliments
8   Salt jars
9   Pool
10 Tasting
11 Knowing your preferences
12 Hangman
13 Just a minute

MOTOR/PHYSICAL ACTIVITIES

14 Circuits
15 Obstacle course
16 Relays

GROUP GAMES

17 Kim's game
18 Spot the differences
19 Mimes
20 Charades
21 Say the picture
22 Who am I?
23 Zoo

WORKING AS A TEAM

24 Making sandwiches
25 Treasure hunt
26 Token challenge
27 Group picnic game

PROBLEM-SOLVING

28 Good and bad things from the week
29 Leaflets/questionnaires
30 Debates
31 Role plays
32 Quizzes
33 Thought showers

EMOTIONS/MENTAL HEALTH

34 Act out emotions
35 Planets
36 Emotional thermometers
37 Life maps
38 Power circles
39 The colour of feelings
40 What's in my head?

List of community visits

A   Beach
B   Café
C   Cinema
D   Going for a pizza
E   Laser quest
F   Public transport
G   Shopping
H   Swimming/Leisure centre
I   Take-away
J   Team games
K   Tenpin bowling

Acknowledgements

We would like to thank the following people for their contributions and support in writing this book:

Carl Ahmed, Peter Conlin, Jill Curry, Susan McBride and Anna Westaway for their helpful comments and positive advice.

Our colleagues and management at South Tyneside Foundation Trust and South Tyneside Primary Care Trust for supporting us in developing our approach and providing the opportunities to try out new initiatives.

Our friends and families for their patience and support during the writing of this book, for reading the book in its various stages, for trying out some of the activities and for giving advice.

Introduction

The authors of this book strongly believe in developing a team approach to working with children who have an Autism Spectrum Disorder (ASD). The book is based on personal experiences. Over several years, we have established a comprehensive and integrated approach to intervention for children with ASD. This includes a programme of groupwork beginning at pre-school (3–5 years) and progressing through the child's school years from primary (5–11 years) to secondary education (11–16 years). This is the final book in a series of three providing a framework for developing groupwork across the age ranges. The content of each book and the recommended groupwork approach are based on the same underlying philosophy, but have been shaped by factors such as the age range of the group members and their level of development. This model of working is the result of a strong desire within our team to share roles and responsibilities for the children and young people we are working with.

We believe that maximum progress can only be achieved when professionals have a holistic view of the young person's strengths and needs and adopt an integrated approach to intervention. Due to the complex needs of young people with ASD and their difficulties generalising newly learned skills into a wide range of settings, working on specific skills in isolation will have limited impact. It is essential to look at all aspects of the young person's development and how they are interlinked in order to plan a logical and co-ordinated approach to developing functional skills and independence. Integrating the knowledge and skills of the multidisciplinary team and using this to set integrated targets for a young person that acknowledge the impact of one developmental area on another is paramount to effective intervention.

Why use groupwork?

As we developed our approach, we became aware of many overlaps in the activities that therapists and other professionals were using. The differences arose in the way that we were analysing the activities, based on our individual professional perspectives. For example, a teacher may be working on personal relationships and sexuality within the educational curriculum in a group setting. At the same time, a clinical psychologist may be addressing issues of self-awareness, acceptance of diagnosis and personal relationships on an individual basis. The young person may be experiencing significant difficulty with the issues being addressed in both settings, but for different reasons. In school, the problems may be related to difficulties with peer interaction or a lack of differentiation in the curriculum. In individual sessions, the young person may be finding it difficult to generalise the individualised work into other settings.

The teacher and clinical psychologist need to integrate their knowledge and expertise. They need to provide a differentiated curriculum that addresses the young person's needs in a graded way; introducing new concepts individually, progressing to small groupwork and finally generalising into everyday situations.

In addition, we found that many of the existing resources targeted only one aspect of a young person's development or were based on one theoretical approach. Few resources exist that highlight the need for this wider analysis of the relationships between different areas of development or the need to link the areas of development together to achieve the ultimate aims of intervention.

Whilst developing the approach, we also acknowledged the heavy commitment required in terms of time for planning, preparation and delivery of the group sessions and individualising the approach to meet the needs of a specific young person. However, we realised that developing a holistic and integrated approach, which addresses all aspects of the young person's presentation in a co-ordinated way, would have many more benefits both for the service user and for the professional team (see Table I).

Feedback from young people, parents and carers

Feedback from young people, parents and carers on this approach has been extremely positive. Some of the comments received from evaluation forms completed by the group members and parents and carers following group sessions have included:

> 'I enjoyed the group because it helped me to learn to look after myself – things like making a cup of tea and a snack. I can make my own dinner when I get home from school now.' (Joe)
>
> 'I didn't see the point of the groups to begin with, but now I think they were really useful. It helped me to understand my diagnosis.' (Lucy)
>
> 'I found it really useful to meet other people with ASD. I am the only person who has ASD in my school and I can feel lonely.' (Omar)
>
> 'It was good to be able to talk about things that are important to me. I could talk to the group about things that were bothering me like my classmates and homework. They had some good ideas to help.' (Philip)
>
> 'After the group finished, Michael was able to go shopping and buy a birthday card for his dad by himself for the first time.' (Parent)
>
> 'I can now trust Penny to get the bus to her grandparents by herself. I just need to walk her to the bus stop and her grandad meets her at the other end.' (Parent)
>
> 'Clare now has a friend to walk home with.' (Carer)
>
> 'You can tell all the kids love coming; it's the highlight of their week.' (Parent)

Advantages of integrated working	Disadvantages of integrated working
• Positive, cross-discipline learning experiences • Shared knowledge and skills, including the interrelationships between areas of development • Increased awareness of each young person's abilities and needs • Consistent and holistic approach to intervention, including joint prioritisation and target setting • Ability to provide the young person and his parent or carer with more manageable targets and achievable expectations • Greater involvement of the young person in planning their own intervention • Improved communication with parents and carers due to increased contact with them • More effective caseload management, eg, seeking initial advice/consultation from another professional rather than making a referral to her • More effective service management, eg, co-ordination of appointments/ periods of intervention	• Time commitment for planning, preparation and running of the group, in particular for individualising approaches and equipment • Resource implications, including maintaining the high staffing ratio

TABLE I Advantages and disadvantages of integrated working identified by the multidisciplinary team

○ Who is the book for?

The book has been compiled by occupational therapists and speech & language therapists but is intended for use by any professionals (particularly those new to the field), support staff, parents and carers working with these young people. We would advise close liaison between all of those involved with the young person and their family to facilitate the assessment process and generalisation of emerging skills across a range of contexts.

Although this book is aimed at a specific age group, it should be used flexibly. For example, a group of young people at the lower end of this age range (11–12 years)

may benefit from some of the activities included in the primary (5–11 years) book. A combination of activities from both resource books would be recommended.

◯ How is the book structured?

The theory

Although a basic awareness of ASD would be helpful, we have included a short theoretical section to provide the knowledge base to explain and support the assessment process and group activities.

The theoretical section begins with a description of autism, including the 'Triad of Impairments' (Wing, 1995). This has been expanded, and its impact on the following areas of development is described:

- Language and communication
- Socialisation
- Leisure time
- Sensory issues
- Motor skills
- Behaviour
- Emotional development

The descriptions of each area are supplemented with examples provided through case studies.

The theoretical section also includes examples of the different models of team working described in the literature and how these relate to our philosophy on integrated working.

The practice

Sections on the importance of assessment (including assessment profiles), keeping records and evaluation are included.

More practical sections follow with information about how to plan and run a group, activities to be used within group sessions and ideas on how to generalise what is learned into community settings.

Towards the end of Chapter 6 we have provided two working examples based on our groups to illustrate the theory, highlight key issues and show the benefits of groupwork. Most readers would find it helpful to read through the working examples to get a real flavour of our integrated approach.

> *It is recommended that readers new to the field of ASD read each section in sequence, but more experienced readers may wish to read the more practical sections only.*

How does the approach work?

Group size

Our aim has been to develop a programme that can be used flexibly to develop skills in a variety of developmental areas, depending on the individual needs of the young person, and in a small group context. We recommend four to six young people as the optimum group size. Maintaining a small group size ensures that the group facilitators develop a detailed knowledge of each young person and have the time required to differentiate activities and personalise the approach to meet individual group members' needs.

The use of assessment

An initial assessment of each young person's individual needs across a number of areas is required. Photocopiable assessment profiles to facilitate this can be found in Chapter 3. This information can be used to set individual targets to focus on during groupwork.

The group sessions

Chapters 4, 5 and 6 provide information on the practicalities of choosing a group, planning and running a group and recording progress. This includes information on consent and risk assessment, who should run the group, choosing your venue, deciding on activities, liaising with parents, carers and professionals, onward referrals, future support needs and what to do when the group does not work.

How the activities help young people with ASD

The activities provided in Chapter 7 are designed to meet young people's needs in the seven key developmental areas:

- Language and communication
- Socialisation
- Leisure time
- Sensory issues
- Motor skills
- Behaviour
- Emotional development

In addition, the following four sub-categories have been used to clarify which aspects of behavioural and emotional development an activity can be used to target when appropriate.

- Understanding of diagnosis
- Transitions
- Self-awareness and the development of coping strategies
- Independent living skills

Each activity can be differentiated according to the area being targeted as well as the individual needs of the young person.

The same activity may be used with one young person to develop a communication skill whilst another young person in the same group is developing understanding of emotions. For example, while creating a thought shower (Activity 33) on bullying, the target for one group member may be to explore the emotions relating to the theme of bullying, whilst another group member may be focusing on conversational skills in a group setting. This prevents overcrowding the session plan with too many activities that are all trying to target something different. This can become confusing for the group facilitators and overwhelming for the young person. A clear and simple session plan with specific but differentiated targets for each young person within an activity is more manageable and effective.

The community visits

Chapter 8 includes suggestions for community visits to plan, complete and evaluate with the group members, particularly those at the facilitating independence stage. All of the skills targeted within group sessions are intended to be functional and generalised into everyday settings. The visits described in Chapter 8 provide a stepping stone to facilitate the generalisation of skills from the group into a supported functional setting before, hopefully, becoming independent living skills requiring minimal levels of support.

Levels of intervention

The activities are graded into levels of intervention, some of which are appropriate for young people at an *emerging independence* stage and some of which are more appropriate for young people at a *facilitating independence* stage of development (see Chapter 7). This enables the group facilitator to select an activity and use it at the appropriate level to meet the young person's identified needs.

Young people working at the emerging independence stage need to develop prerequisite skills with higher levels of adult support. For example, a young person may work on recognising coins and money management in the group setting before being expected to apply these skills on a shopping trip.

Young people working at the facilitating independence stage will have acquired many of the prerequisite skills and will be working on applying these into a community setting with gradually reducing levels of support.

The grading of activities enables the group facilitators to simplify or extend the activity for a young person, depending on how well they perform the task and their level of independence. It also enables the group members to work at different levels to each other whilst still sharing an activity. The group facilitators need to be very clear about the level they expect each young person to achieve within an activity and the level of support required in order to ensure they succeed.

The format of the activities

The activities are designed to be used creatively and flexibly. They can be modified to meet the needs of a variety of young people and to suit different group contexts. The targets we have given for each activity are not exhaustive and can be adapted to meet your own group members' needs.

All of the activities include:

 A list of the equipment required (suppliers' details are provided in Appendix XXV)

 Examples of individual targets that the activities could be used to meet

 Top tips that give helpful information on running the group as effectively as possible

 Instructions on how to carry out the activities (graded into different levels)

Where appropriate, we have also included:

 A cautionary note to remind group facilitators to be aware of potential emotional/mental health concerns within an activity, which may need careful handling. This not only relates to the emotional/mental health status of the young person, but also to the group facilitator's confidence and competence to carry out these activities. It may be more appropriate for professionals new to the field of ASD to refer to a more experienced colleague.

A detailed list of all the activities in the book is provided in Chapter 7 and suggestions for community visits in Chapter 8.

Using the activities in a group session

The emphasis throughout the activities is on developing functional communication and teaching skills important for the activities of daily living with increasing opportunities for developing independence. As a result, the session plan for a group in this age range should be extremely flexible and responsive to the needs of the individual group members at any given time.

For the younger end of this age range (11–13 years), we would suggest a basic session structure as follows:

- Warm-up activity
- 2–3 activities
- Snack time
- 2–3 activities
- Round-up activity

This should be reviewed at the start of the group session with the group members, and then after the session with the group facilitators as part of the peer review process. Modifications suggested after the peer review can be implemented at the start of the next group session.

For the older end of the age range (14–16 years), we would recommend a more open session structure. Group facilitators should create a rough session plan, but this should be discussed and negotiated with the group prior to the session starting and adapted according to their needs and preferences. This encourages the group members to take responsibility for identifying their own needs, setting their own targets and planning how to meet these needs.

Resources

The final sections of the book include photocopiable handouts to help in the planning, preparation and evaluation of your group (see Appendices I–XXVI).

Readers may find the suggestions for the contents of a collage box (Appendix VII), sensory box (Appendix XX) and the list of suppliers (Appendix XXV) at the end of the book particularly useful in building up a resource base for use within the group.

We have also included a recommended reading list for any readers who wish to find out more about any specific aspects of our work.

What is Autism Spectrum Disorder?

Autism was first described by Kanner in 1943 (Aarons & Gittens, 1992). Frith (1991) highlighted the work of Hans Asperger, who described a similar disorder, but with differing levels of impairment. The difficulties he described later became known as Asperger's Syndrome. Over the years, interest in these disorders has varied, with a recent resurgence of interest in what is now commonly referred to as Autism Spectrum Disorder (ASD). This describes a spectrum of difficulties with shared core deficits that may present in a variety of ways.

Diagnosis and classification of ASD is a complex and detailed process, which will not be described in this book. Clinicians involved in diagnosis will usually use well-recognised criteria such as DSM IV (American Psychiatric Association, 1994) or ICD-10 (World Health Organisation, 1993). These enable clinicians to map an individual's presentation and attribute a diagnostic label, where appropriate, according to national and local guidelines.

Whilst a diagnostic label may have some benefits, it does not provide a description of a young person's strengths and needs. For professionals working directly with these young people, it is important to understand the underlying reasons for differences in their presentation. This enables more effective educational and therapeutic interventions to be identified.

Wing (1995) described the difficulties experienced in ASD as a 'Triad of Impairments'. This is a useful way to describe the complex patterns of behaviour presented. This model recognises that behaviour, thinking and learning styles are influenced by fundamental differences in the development of communication, socialisation skills and limited flexibility in imagination. It is this model that we have used when thinking about the needs of our client group.

In our experience, in addition to the three main areas of impairment, there are a number of young people with ASD who also have significant motor and sensory difficulties. For this reason, we have added these to the model to provide a more comprehensive representation of the difficulties experienced (see Figure 1.1).

Whilst diagnosis is based on a pattern of behaviours that are the result of these common core deficits, each young person's presentation is unique. A young person's developmental profile will show areas of relative strength alongside areas of specific need. This diversity has fostered the use of the term 'spectrum' to describe this disorder, as no two people with ASD are alike.

Differences in these five areas may have a profound affect on a young person's progress in all aspects of his development. The young person with ASD may differ significantly from his peers in many ways. In our experience, difficulties are often reported within the seven areas of development described below.

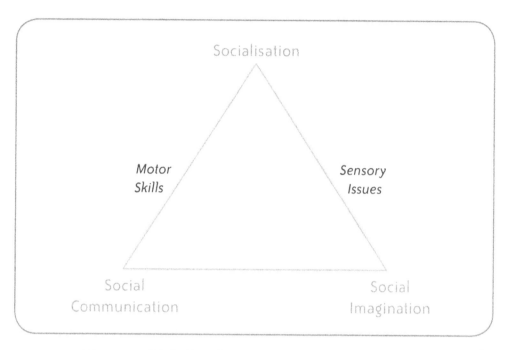

FIGURE 1.1 'Triad of Impairments'. Adapted from Wing L, 1995, *Autistic Spectrum Disorders: An Aid to Diagnosis*, p5, National Autistic Society, London. Reproduced with permission.

◯ Language and communication

Difficulties with language and communication are central to ASD, but they manifest in many different ways. In the 3–5 age range, many children we work with remain at a non-intentional phase of communication or intentional communication is only just beginning to emerge. The emphasis with this younger age group is, therefore, on establishing communication in any form rather than on developing specific spoken language skills.

By school age, however, basic communication skills in group members are generally well-established and the emphasis changes to working on more specific spoken language or functional communication skills (eg, describing, explaining or disagreeing in an appropriate and effective way).

The pattern of language development in children and young people with ASD is frequently disordered or deviates from the typical pattern seen in other young people, but the profile for each young person with ASD will be unique.

In our experience, difficulties in the following areas are frequently seen, and these will impact on the young person's functional communication and ability to engage in everyday situations.

Poor attention and listening

Many young people with ASD may present as easily distracted or lacking the ability to focus their attention. Attention and listening difficulties may have a sensory basis. Some young people may experience difficulties with auditory information (spoken words, pitch and intonation) whilst others may experience difficulty with visual information (facial expressions and gestures). The impact can be far-reaching and affect the ability to register and interpret verbal and non-verbal communication.

Others may experience difficulties resulting from overloading of the sensory systems (eg, the classroom is too noisy or they feel uncomfortable due to tags on clothing). Difficulties in modulating or inhibiting sensory input can make it impossible to focus attention on more appropriate or important aspects of their environment.

CASE STUDY

SUSAN is 12 years old, with a diagnosis of ASD. She coped well in her small local primary school, but has recently transferred to a much bigger comprehensive school. Her teacher has noticed that she is having considerable difficulty concentrating in the classroom due to the increased class size, noisier environment and the requirement to work independently for greater amounts of time. A number of strategies were introduced to improve her attention and listening skills, including seating her at the front of the class to focus her attention on the teacher and providing one-to-one support when available. In addition, factors to reduce noise levels within the classroom were identified, for example, ensuring the door is closed to minimise corridor noise, seating her away from noise-making equipment and loud peers.

Poor auditory memory

Many young people with ASD have difficulty retaining information that has been given verbally.

Some young people have problems with auditory sequential memory (ie, remembering a list of items), resulting in an inability to remember shopping lists, telephone numbers or to follow sequences of instructions. For example, an instruction given in the classroom such as 'You need to finish reading Chapter 1, answer the questions on page 10, then hand your workbook in to be marked' may cause difficulties because the young person cannot remember everything on the list.

Some young people may experience difficulties with working memory (ie, holding information in the memory whilst acting upon it). These young people may experience problems remembering sequences of instructions in cookery or science lessons, for example, where there is an expectation to recall information whilst continuing to follow a recipe or complete an experiment.

Some young people can remember information immediately after it is given, but cannot recall it after a prolonged period (long-term memory). These young people may need frequent reminders of things that they have been told many times before. A common theme that we have come across is problems with remembering and completing homework.

Auditory memory problems of any kind are greatly facilitated by the use of visual helpers.

CASE STUDY

BRIAN is 13 years old, with a diagnosis of ASD. He is frequently in trouble for not completing and returning his homework. He is often given detention as a result of this. His problems were identified as being the result of poor long-term memory. A homework diary was introduced in which Brian was encouraged to record his homework assignments at the end of each lesson. Providing him with this visual helper to remind him of his homework, including what to do and when to hand it in, resulted in more consistent completion and return of his work and fewer detentions.

Understanding of language

Whilst young people with ASD may present with a wide range of receptive language difficulties, some features tend to be common to this group. They include difficulty with:

- Prepositions (for example, 'between', 'above', 'below')
- Pronouns (for example, 'his'/'her'/'their')
- Understanding question words (for example, 'who?', 'where?', 'why?')
- Understanding vocabulary associated with time/sequence (for example, 'last week', 'yesterday', 'in a minute')
- Understanding language associated with emotions (for example, 'angry', 'proud', 'surprised')

Many young people with ASD interpret language in a very literal or concrete way. These young people will experience difficulties in understanding the subtleties of language, such as ambiguity, humour, metaphors, idioms, sarcasm or irony. Difficulty with these high-level language skills means that they will have problems in drawing inferences and making predictions. Using language to facilitate mental processes such as reasoning and problem-solving will also be impaired.

CASE STUDY

SHAFIQ is 15 years old, with a diagnosis of Asperger's Syndrome. He has a very literal understanding of language that results in many social faux pas. For example, he has recently become interested in girls and would like to have a girlfriend. However, he has found it difficult to establish a relationship due to his lack of understanding of rhetorical questions. In a recent conversation with a female peer, she asked him if he thought she had put weight on. Not realising that she did not want to hear the truthful answer, he replied honestly with 'yes'! This caused great offence and resulted in a breakdown in their friendship. Shafiq struggled to understand why his comments had caused such a reaction. The concept of rhetorical questions and the use of ambiguity were discussed within a group session and appropriate responses explored through role play to help him to cope more successfully in similar situations in the future.

Expressive language

Some young people with ASD will have difficulties with expressive language, similar to the problematic areas in the understanding of language (eg, an inability to use the appropriate preposition). Others will use language that they have learnt from others without fully understanding what it means. This can mask underlying difficulties with understanding. People may assume that, as the young people can use complex language, they must understand it and so they place too high expectations upon them.

Common difficulties in the area of expressive language may include:

Word-finding difficulties

Some young people with ASD have problems in recalling vocabulary for use at the time when it is needed. Young people may use a word in one context, but then struggle to recall it for use in another. This may be the result of a faulty 'filing system' associated with poor auditory memory. The young person with word-finding difficulties may have long gaps or pauses in his conversation as he struggles to find the word he needs. He may use the same familiar and well-learned vocabulary over and over again, giving his speech a repetitive quality. Alternatively, he may use another word with a similar meaning, making his expressive language slightly odd or inappropriate in nature. Young people with word-finding problems may fail to make the links between associated words and their meanings and this can affect their ability to make predictions, draw inferences and solve problems.

Sequencing

Difficulties with organisation and sequencing are apparent in many aspects of the young person's development, and language is no exception. Word-finding difficulties can impact on the young person's ability to generate an idea and sequence words in a logical way to express himself appropriately and effectively. Sequencing problems may result in the young person using sentences with confused word order or inappropriate structure. They may result in the use of 'fillers' to hold the floor while the young person organises his thoughts during conversation. It may present as a problem with fluency as the young person stops and starts his sentence a number of times before getting it right.

Alternatively, it can affect his ability to order a longer narrative or retell a story. The order of occurrence of events may become confused, so that a narrative or story does not flow or make sense.

Social use of language

Even when language skills appear to be reasonably well-established, most young people with ASD experience difficulties in how they use their language in a social setting.

Language is used purposefully for a variety of functions, including to:

- Attract attention
- Make choices or requests
- Refuse or reject something
- Ask questions
- Answer questions
- Comment
- Direct
- Be sociable

In most children, these skills are established within the first 12 months of life and emerge in parallel. In young people with ASD, these functional uses of language may need to be actively taught by parents, carers and professionals. They tend to appear one-by-one and over a very long time period and differ according to the young person's experiences. Often, these skills may not be fully established even in the late school years or early adulthood. These young people may experience significant difficulty in using language to enable them to cope or function in everyday situations that require negotiating skills, finding appropriate ways to disagree or criticise, giving praise or compliments or seeking help and clarification.

The areas of language and communication that can be affected in young people with ASD are wide-ranging and can have a major impact on the young person's ability to function successfully in a variety of areas, including socialisation, leisure time, behaviour and emotional development.

CASE STUDY

BEN is 14 years old and has a diagnosis of ASD. In formal assessment situations, his expressive language skills appear to be very good. However, in everyday situations he tends to be very quiet and withdrawn. This is the result of poor generalisation of expressive language skills and an inability to use his language for social functions. For example, he rarely initiates interaction as he has no strategies for opening a conversation. The group facilitators worked on asking social questions using interviews (Activity 3) to teach him how to use his expressive language skills for a social function.

Socialisation

As young people progress through the education system, the demands on social understanding and for them to engage in appropriate social interactions increase dramatically. Parents and carers or siblings may have previously acted as the main interface between the young person and the outside world. Their ability to facilitate in this way decreases as the young person enters into early adolescence where there are increasing expectations to move towards independence. We have found there is generally an increase in awareness (in both the young people themselves and/or those around them) of the differences in the ways in which these young people engage socially in comparison with their peers at this time.

The most significant difference is the motivation to engage with others for social purposes. Young people with ASD generally fall into one of two groups. The first is the 'unmotivated' group, who are often described as 'in a world of their own' or not interested in other people. The second group are the 'socially motivated' young people, who want to interact but use inappropriate ways to make social contact.

The difficulties that the young person experiences may be explained by some underlying differences in development, such as:

Shared attention

By the age of 11, many young people have developed some ability for shared attention, but often it is qualitatively different from the rest of their peers. At one extreme, there may be young people who can engage in shared attention when it is expected of them (eg, during one-to-one tasks in the classroom) but choose not to initiate shared attention at other times. These young people may have developed special interests or sensory-seeking or stereotypical behaviours that they would choose to engage in to the exclusion of all others.

Others may be extremely motivated to share their interests with their peers and initiate shared attention in order to do so. However, due to their difficulties with recognising and interpreting non-verbal cues (such as facial expressions), they may lack awareness of when their listener has lost interest or become confused, or when it is inappropriate to say things (eg, talking loudly in a quiet classroom or talking about private matters in a public place). These young people will find it difficult to monitor a situation and change their language and behaviour to suit the context and, although keen to be 'one of the crowd', are often excluded as a result.

CASE STUDY

HUSSEIN is 11 years old, with a diagnosis of ASD. He is very sociable and wants to make friends with his peers. However, he tends to be very loud and boisterous, which draws attention to him and anyone in close proximity. As a result, many of his peers have started to avoid him. The group facilitators worked on his non-verbal communication skills, in particular speech volume and proximity to others, using friendship darts (Activity 6) and role plays (Activity 31) to teach him more socially acceptable ways of initiating and maintaining friendships with his peers.

Understanding facial expression and body language

A young person with ASD tends to decode information in small parts and may be very interested in detail rather than whole experiences. He may, for example, focus on a person's moving lips when they are talking, rather than considering the whole facial expression and associated body language. In addition, he may not understand emotions or that other people are not experiencing things exactly as he does. This is described by Frith (1991) as difficulties with 'Theory of Mind'. The young person may therefore misinterpret a person's presentation or misread a situation due to a lack of awareness of non-verbal means of communicating, limited understanding of emotions and an inability to recognise differing perspectives.

These differences explain why the young person may show unusual social behaviours that are inappropriate to the context (eg, laughing at sad news). It also explains why it usually takes a young person with ASD longer to learn social rules and conventions, to understand social boundaries and to learn to function independently in everyday situations.

○ Leisure time

In our experience, leisure activities take up a large proportion of an adolescent's time and we feel it is therefore important that they have a sense of control over how they spend this time. Friends and the social environment play a central role in developing a sense of belonging. However, in our experience, young people with ASD often show differences in how they use their leisure time.

Many young people continue to display areas of special interest. These are often related to their sensory preferences, learning styles and/or limitations in flexibility of thinking or imagination described in the 'Triad of Impairments' (see Figure 1.1). These young people are often good at learning facts and figures and, as a result, interests often involve grouping, ordering and systematisation. Some of the young people we have worked with have been interested in computers, transport and the solar system, for example, but special interests can be very private, idiosyncratic and time-consuming. Their motivation to engage with activities outside their area of interest can be low and therefore leisure opportunities become limited.

Some young people with ASD may be willing to experience a wider range of leisure activities but rely on their parents or carers to manage their leisure time. This may be for a number of reasons. For example, some parents and carers may be reluctant to allow their child out alone due to their sensory sensitivities, language and communication difficulties or social vulnerability. These young people are not in control of their own leisure time and may struggle with developing a sense of belonging.

The development of greater independence and the transition into adulthood can have emotional and psychosocial effects on the young person and require consideration from all the professionals involved with them.

Within an intervention programme, it is often advisable to incorporate supported leisure opportunities as an objective, with graded phasing out of support to semi-directed and then (where possible) fully independent leisure time.

CASE STUDY

PHILIP is 16 years old, with a diagnosis of Asperger's Syndrome. He has a special interest in Formula One cars and car racing. He will sit for many hours looking at car magazines, searching the internet for cars and talking to people about the make, model and specifications of their car. His interest was all-consuming and interfered with his motivation to engage in alternative leisure activities. The group facilitators used his special interest to encourage him to try out new activities. For example, he was encouraged to go to the shop to buy his car magazines, rather than his parents buying them for him. He was also persuaded to go to the bowling alley with friends where there was a car-racing arcade game to practise taking turns with his peers.

Sensory issues

In Sensory Integration theory (Bundy *et al*, 2002) there are seven recognisable senses:

- Auditory (hearing)
- Visual (sight)
- Gustatory (taste)
- Olfactory (smell)
- Tactile (touch)
- Proprioception (movement – receptors in the muscles and joints provide us with a sense of body awareness)
- Vestibular (balance – receptors in the inner ear send messages to the brain to enable us to maintain posture, balance and motor control)

More information on this can be found on the Sensory Integration website (www. sensoryintegration.org.uk).

In our experience, people with ASD may have different sensory experiences from their peers without ASD. Almost all of the young people that we work with have some sensory issues that impact on their behaviour, communication and ability to engage in social interactions.

Thresholds

Dunn (1999) developed a tool to assist in understanding sensory behaviours and relates this to a framework that can be the basis for providing therapeutic and environmental interventions. Dunn describes behaviours in terms of thresholds (high versus low).

Thresholds in any system relate to how much sensory information the system needs to respond. A high threshold means the system needs a high level of input to make a response. A low threshold means the system needs only a little input to make a response.

A *high threshold* in any sense elicits one of two types of behaviour:

Sensory seeking

A young person with a high threshold for auditory input may need to constantly listen to music on his MP3 player in order to concentrate.

Poor registration

A young person with a high threshold for auditory input may not register when spoken to in a voice at normal volume.

Similarly, a *low threshold* elicits one of two behaviours:

Avoidance

A young person with a low threshold for auditory input will avoid situations where there are loud noises, such as discos or shops.

Sensitivity

A young person with a low threshold for auditory input may cover his ears (eg, with a hat or hoodie) in noisy environments such as shops.

Almost all behaviours that we are presented with could have a sensory origin. Using this knowledge, we can begin to find ways in which we can assist young people with ASD to develop awareness of and articulate their thresholds, give strategies to help them to manage their environment and offer techniques to provide their level of sensory needs in an appropriate and organised way.

> CASE STUDY
>
> **KIN** is 13 years old, with a diagnosis of ASD. He has a high threshold for movement (proprioception) and constantly seeks high levels of activity (e.g. shuffling on his chair, being unable to stand still in queues, being extremely boisterous during physical activities such as PE). The group facilitators adapted the structure of the group to include regular controlled movement breaks, which enabled Kin to concentrate more fully during table-top activities. These included giving out equipment, making the drinks, being the timetable monitor and helping to move furniture before the obstacle course.

○ Motor skills

Young people with ASD may have experienced difficulties with balance and co-ordination throughout life resulting in, for example, never being picked for the team, failure to succeed at sports day and clumsiness during everyday activities. These negative experiences, which may be combined with a lack of social drive to fit in with their peers, may further impact on motivation to try new tasks and develop skills.

Between the ages of 11 and 16, these difficulties may significantly impact on a young person's ability to develop independent living skills. Everyday activities such as making a cup of tea, cooking a simple meal or doing the washing up may be extremely difficult for them and will impact on this person's ability to function without support and may also limit their social opportunities. For example, some young people with ASD may avoid joining youth clubs that require them to help with tasks such as setting up the room, making snacks and washing up.

> CASE STUDY
>
> **MARTIN** is 16 years old, with a diagnosis of autism. He has a significant motor-planning problem. Many of his peers at school are joining the gym, but he is reluctant to go with them because he is afraid that he will be laughed at for being so clumsy. The group facilitators and the group members identified activities to develop motor-planning skills using circuits (Activity 14, Level 5) and agreed to work towards a group trip to the gym as a community visit. Whilst Martin's motor skills did not significantly improve over the course of the group, he developed greater self-confidence and willingness to attend a gym with support, working towards independent access.

○ Behaviour

At times, all of us display behaviours that could be described as difficult. During adolescence, in particular, there are changes in the behaviour of many young people, relating to hormonal changes, the desire to be socially accepted and/or anxiety due to exam pressures, for example. Also, the onset of puberty can lead to issues relating to sexuality, sexual relationships and behaviour. In addition to all of these, young people with ASD may have to cope with repeated failure, negative experiences and an increasing awareness of their differences.

The approaches used to address difficult behaviour in others will often not work with young people with ASD. There are a number of reasons for this.

Social motivation

Most of us have an understanding of the world as a social setting where there are expectations and social norms (eg, not making personal comments in public places). A young person with ASD may have little understanding of these concepts or of another person's thoughts and feelings and therefore is unlikely to be motivated by pleasing others.

Sensory behaviours and thresholds

Many of the behaviours that we observe may have a sensory basis and can be interpreted as a need rather than a difficult behaviour. Often, a purely behavioural approach to managing these behaviours will only result in another, often more inappropriate behaviour, replacing it. For example, preventing a young person from using a large piece of silky material to stroke for comfort may result in the development of a more inappropriate behaviour such as seeking other materials to feel (eg, stroking someone's hair or clothing). It is more appropriate to encourage a more discreetly sized piece of silky material being kept in the pocket and used when required by the young person.

Lack of understanding

The young person with ASD may not have the cognitive or linguistic skills to understand verbal instructions and therefore may not learn or understand consequences as others do.

Generalisation

A young person with ASD often has great difficult in generalising information. He may learn not to swear at his head teacher but will see swearing at the science teacher as a completely different situation.

Development of coping strategies

Many young people with ASD have experienced ongoing difficulties in educational and social situations (eg, bullying, auditory overload or social isolation). As a result, they have developed a wide range of coping strategies. Some of these may be highly appropriate, but in our experience many are complex and elaborate behaviours that are used to avoid or disrupt situations where difficulties are anticipated. These behaviours, however negative they appear to us, enable the young person to maintain a degree of control and predictability over a situation (eg, 'If I swear at the teacher, I'll be removed from the classroom and won't have to do this work'). Therefore, from their perspective, they have a positive outcome.

Transitions

The transition from childhood to adulthood brings with it many challenges for the young person with ASD and their parents or carers. The educational environment changes, as the movement between classrooms and changing peer groups, subjects and teachers becomes a daily requirement. At various stages, there is the transition between year groups and the need to choose courses, with exams bringing yet more changes to the daily timetable. Ultimately, there is the transition from the educational sector into the adult world and the requirement to make decisions about further education or work.

Each of these transitions raises new challenges for the young person with ASD. The emotional impact and behavioural responses may be significant and will require constant monitoring and management by the professionals working with the young person.

○ Emotional development

Emotional stress is a concern many young people and their parents highlight as an issue in the 11–16 age group. As young people increase their social networks and are more susceptible to the views of others, some are able to perceive the disapproval and rejection that result from their differences.

These young people will require support in understanding their diagnosis and the long-term implications. Many may have low self-esteem, a feeling that they are different and frustration at their inability to 'get it right'. A number of young people may also develop more significant mental health issues (eg, depression or psychosis) that require referral to a mental health team.

Although these are also issues for a large number of adolescents, the way to deal with them in a young person with ASD differs. The young person may not be able to discuss things on an emotional level due to poor understanding of these concepts. A more cognitive and behavioural method is used as this approach is less abstract and more practical for the young person with ASD.

CASE STUDIES

DAVID is 15 years old, with a diagnosis of Asperger's Syndrome. He has been experiencing increasing levels of anxiety in relation to his exams and has a fear of failure and his future prospects. On several occasions, he has experienced panic attacks within the school setting and has had to be brought home due to his distressed state. The group facilitators used emotional thermometers (Activity 36, Level 2) and What's in my head? (Activity 40, Level 2) to explore his feelings and discuss coping strategies. In addition, he was referred to the child and adolescent psychiatrist to consider any medical interventions that may be helpful.

LEELA is 13 years old, with a diagnosis of ASD. Her eating habits have changed dramatically since a lesson in school about nutrition and healthy diet. As a result, she has established a concrete belief system around 'good' and 'bad' food. She refuses to eat anything that she considers 'bad' food and believes that people who do eat these foods must be 'bad' people. She was referred to a clinical psychologist to address these issues using cognitive and behavioural approaches as she was unable to discuss her beliefs due to limited understanding of the emotional concepts required within the group.

Encouraging young people to participate actively in groupwork provides an opportunity to engage them in exploring their strengths and needs in relation to their diagnosis as well as in developing essential strategies to cope with everyday experiences.

Groupwork enables young people to share knowledge and experiences with each other, to share strategies to develop their skills and reduce inappropriate behaviours, and it also offers emotional support. This information can, with their consent, be shared with parents and carers to help the family as a unit to support one another.

We hope that by intervening in this way and including the young person in the process, they can develop the skills required to deal with a challenging world.

Working in a team

ASD is a pervasive developmental disorder affecting all aspects of a young person's development. These differences in development may have a significant impact on every aspect of their life, for example, on personal relationships, leisure activities and the activities of daily living. As a result, the young person and his family often find that a huge array of professionals become involved in the assessment and diagnostic process and intervention, and at times this can feel overwhelming.

These professionals may be from the health, education, social care, independent or voluntary sectors. The agencies that they represent frequently differ in organisational structure and administration systems. The professionals have been through different training routes and have different priorities. In our experience, this can be very confusing for the young person and his family for a number of reasons. These may include lack of clarity over professionals' roles, repetition of assessments, lack of co-ordination in the timing of various aspects of the assessment, poor liaison over educational and therapeutic interventions, and differences in the use and understanding of terminology.

All of those working with the young person with ASD are part of a team. It is only by working as a team that we can achieve the best results for these young people. Although this book is written by occupational therapists and speech & language therapists, it is intended for use by any member of the team, including therapists, teachers, nursing staff, psychologists, support staff, parents and carers.

> *We would recommend that the group facilitators, whatever their background, liaise with other key people in the young person's life. This ensures that an accurate assessment of the young person is achieved, and that there is consistency in the areas of development targeted and in the approaches being used.*

Who are the key members of the team?

This section summarises the key team members, based on our experiences, but we acknowledge that team membership and roles vary enormously in different localities.

The make-up of the team will vary according to locality, resources, national and local policy and the individual needs of the young person and his family. Most areas have a local directory that lists the available services and will help you to identify the key professionals in your own team.

The young person with ASD

Many young people at this age are very aware of their strengths and differences, and possibly their diagnosis. It is essential to involve the young person as much as possible in identifying his own needs and the most appropriate strategies to manage them. Failing to include the young person may lead to a lack of motivation towards interventions or the development of inappropriate coping or avoidance strategies. Ultimately, therefore, any intervention provided will not be effective.

Parents and carers

The parents and carers are the constant presence in a young person's life and, as such, the link between all of the professionals and support staff involved with the young person. Parents and carers have the greatest interest in and motivation to help their child and are, without doubt, one of the most important members of the team.

The occupational therapist

The occupational therapist understands how differences in development impact on leisure time and interests, behaviour, emotions and the activities of daily living. Her emphasis is on the young person's ability to understand his environment, perform everyday skills (eg, dressing, making meals or integrating into the community) and function in everyday situations. In particular, the occupational therapist will analyse a young person's sensory processing and motor skills in relation to independent functioning.

What will their assessment involve?

The occupational therapist's assessment is likely to involve collecting information from the young person, his parents or carers and other professionals, alongside observation of him in a range of everyday situations. Some standardised assessments may be used to assess specific aspects of his development and the young person's opinions may also be sought using self-rating scales, for example.

A profile of the young person's strengths and needs is created. This will enable the occupational therapist to formulate a management plan that may include activities to develop leisure skills, sensory integration, motor skills and to address any self-esteem or mental health issues. Her emphasis is on developing functional skills that can be broken down into small, achievable steps.

The speech & language therapist

The speech & language therapist looks at a young person's speech, language and communication skills. In particular, the speech & language therapist will assess attention and listening skills, understanding and expressive language, high-level language skills, intelligibility and the young person's social awareness and interaction skills.

What will their assessment involve?

The speech & language therapist's assessment is likely to be based on information provided by the young person, his parents or carers and other professionals, alongside observation of him in a variety of social settings. A range of standardised assessments may be used and self-rating scales completed by the young person. A profile of his strengths and needs is created, which enables the speech & language therapist to identify a management plan.

The speech & language therapist may focus on strategies to cope with and develop attention and listening skills, difficulties with understanding and expressive language and social awareness and interaction skills.

Other health professionals

The *community/school nurse* or *health visitor* may identify concerns about a young person's development and make onward referrals. Their role is to promote mental, physical and social wellbeing by giving advice, support and practical help to him and his family.

Learning disability/mental health nurses or *family therapists* may have a similar role, working with the young person and family to promote health and wellbeing. Some may work directly with the young person to develop specific skills, whilst others may work through parents and carers offering advice, counselling and support. The issues arising will vary between families and within families at different stages of the young person's life. These may include, for example, managing relationships, developing coping strategies and understanding the diagnosis of ASD.

The *paediatrician* may be involved in providing medical advice or intervention where appropriate. A *psychiatrist* may also be involved to address mental health issues or monitor medical interventions. The paediatrician or psychiatrist may be the lead health professional responsible for co-ordination of health services.

A *clinical psychologist* may be involved with some young people to analyse development and behaviour, consider the impact of wider social and psychological issues and provide practical strategies for managing difficult situations.

Other health professionals who may be involved include a dietician, physiotherapist, osteopath, chiropractor or homeopath. There will be huge variation, depending on the individual needs of the young person and his family.

Education professionals

Most young people at this age will still be in some form of education. This may be a mainstream school, special school, resourced unit or home education programme.

There is now a greater emphasis placed on the role of schools in promoting the health and wellbeing of children and young people, alongside colleagues from other organisations such as social care and health. Professionals from all these organisations must work in partnership in the provision of services for children and young people and their families, leading towards more integrated service delivery (eg, joint group facilitation by teachers and therapists). This is quite different from how services may have been delivered historically, where professionals and organisations often had quite distinct and segregated roles and responsibilities (eg, teachers delivered the educational curriculum and therapists focused on community or life skills without considering how the two could be linked together).

Every Child Matters (DfES, 2003) sets out five key outcomes for children that schools and their partner organisations must work towards:

- **being healthy:** enjoying good physical and mental health and living a healthy lifestyle
- **staying safe:** being protected from harm and neglect
- **enjoying and achieving:** getting the most out of life and developing the skills for adulthood
- **making a positive contribution:** being involved with the community and society and not engaging in anti-social or offending behaviour
- **economic well-being:** not being prevented by economic disadvantage from achieving their full potential in life.

Every Child Matters: Summary of Green Paper, p7. © Crown Copyright 2003. Reproduced under the terms of the Click-Use Licence.

The *teacher* and *education support team* (eg, learning support assistant and educational psychologist) working with the young person play a significant role in his life at this age. Many of the skills that a young person with ASD needs to achieve would fall within one or more of the key outcomes. The school setting will be a key learning environment for many young people targeted within the groupwork model we are proposing. Close liaison between the group facilitators and professionals in the education system is extremely important to ensure that the educational curriculum and these important life skills are brought together to provide a seamless and consistent learning environment for the young person.

Every Child Matters proposes that achieving good outcomes for these young people will be facilitated by working in partnership and through effective integration of services and workforce reform.

The model of working that we propose for the planning, preparation and running of the groups (see below) will, hopefully, provide schools and their partner agencies with a useful tool in meeting the needs of young people with ASD in a co-ordinated and integrated way.

At this stage, some young people may be seeking advice from *transition advisors* and *careers services*. These services will help the young person to make plans with regards to future educational placements, employment or further training.

Social care professionals

Some families, depending on circumstance, may also have access to a *social worker*, *respite care* or *outreach worker* who is responsible for providing access to leisure and social activities as well as providing support for the young person and his family as a whole.

The independent and voluntary sector

A range of independent and voluntary sector services are emerging, which provide a variety of activities for young people with ASD and their families. These may include educational programmes, therapy programmes and outreach or respite care.

Other agencies

Language disorders are a key feature of ASD (see Chapter 1). Clegg *et al*, (1999) describe the persisting difficulties that children with language disorders experience in adolescence and adult life. Their study shows that many of these young people experience residual and/or persisting difficulties in the following areas:

- Mental health problems
- A lack of employment opportunities
- A lack of financial independence
- A lack of independent living – many continue to reside in the parental home, causing familial stress
- Poor social functioning and integration into mainstream services and facilities
- A lack of consistent, multidisciplinary support from professional services

As a result, these young people are at greater risk of psychiatric problems and/or involvement with the police and judicial system.

Some young people may therefore need the support and advice of local *mental health* or *psychiatric services* and/or the local *youth offending team*.

It is important to be aware of the wider range of professionals that may be involved with adolescents and young adults and to ensure that liaison extends to these specialist services.

○ The importance of teamwork

The young person with ASD shows differences in his thinking and learning. This may lead to him performing a skill once and not trying again or learning a skill in one specific context but being unable to generalise into other similar situations. The benefit of teamworking is that it maximises the opportunities for generalisation of skills as all team members are working towards a common set of aims.

In addition, each area is intrinsically linked with others, so that progress in one area is dependent on progress in another. For example, if a young person has emotional/mental health issues, these are likely to impact on his ability to socialise and interact with peers and the environment. However, progress with socialisation targets is likely to be limited unless the underlying emotional/mental health issues are also targeted.

Individual professionals working in isolation, perhaps even using different approaches, will result in the young person developing superficial skills which are of little functional use. In the above example, the mental health professional and speech & language therapist need to work together and develop an approach that targets all relevant developmental areas as a whole. For the young person to maximise his potential, a holistic and integrated approach to intervention needs to be developed.

○ Models of teamworking

Several models of teamworking have been described (Wright & Kersner, 1998; Kashman & Mora, 2002; Watson *et al*, 2002). The literature suggests that a continuum exists, where the main differences relate to the relationships between professionals within the team, as described in this section. All of the figures used below are our own representation of the models listed.

The consultation model

The consultation model (Wright & Kersner, 1998) involves an 'expert' giving advice or recommendations to another person who plays only a participatory role in this relationship. We feel that this approach creates a hierarchy and a dependency that is undesirable in a working partnership.

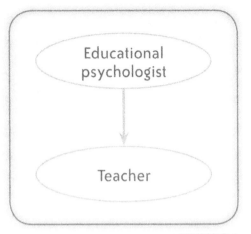

FIGURE 2.1

A representation of the relationship within a consultation model

EXAMPLE

An educational psychologist provides a behaviour modification programme for a young person, to be carried out by the teacher on a daily basis in the school setting. The programme is reviewed and modified by the educational psychologist at regular intervals. The educational psychologist is perceived to be the 'expert' with the knowledge and skills to set behavioural targets and devise a programme to modify behaviour. The programme is given to the teacher but the knowledge and skills underpinning the programme are not shared and the educational psychologist retains the position of 'expert practitioner'.

This consultation model has several disadvantages. Firstly, the maintenance of an 'expert practitioner' means that those actually carrying out the programme may have limited understanding of what they are doing, how to do it and why they are doing it. This means that, if the young person is experiencing difficulties, the programme cannot be simplified or, conversely, if the young person achieves the targets set for him, the expectations cannot be expanded without consulting the 'expert practitioner'. This may result in activities being incorrectly carried out or time delays, as arrangements are made for the 'expert practitioner' to review the situation. As a result, the young person may be unable to practise newly emerging skills consistently or at an appropriate level to suit his changing or developing needs.

Secondly, the 'expert practitioner' may be unaware of the actual needs of the young person in terms of day-to-day, functional skills. She may prioritise skills that will have limited functional benefit and be unaware of the needs within the curriculum and the classroom environment.

Thirdly, the provision of a specific programme of activities may lead to isolated learning. Setting aside time each day to carry out the programme is important, but for young people with ASD there must be a focus on generalisation of skills into functional, everyday situations. Therefore, the adult working with them needs to understand the ultimate aims of the programme. For example, a young person may have a programme that aims to reduce inappropriate behaviour in a class group situation, such as shouting out and invading people's personal space. Following the programme without consideration of how to transfer these skills into other, everyday situations (such as the after-school club) will result in improved behaviours failing to generalise. Therefore, the adult working with the young person needs to be given the knowledge and skills to encourage generalisation of skills so that positive behaviours can be integrated into everyday settings as well.

The collaboration model

The collaboration model (Wright & Kersner, 1998) is probably the most commonly occurring approach, where professionals liaise and share information to solve problems together. Although a sharing relationship, each individual professional brings different strengths and expertise and may or may not jointly implement their agreed goals.

| Educational psychologist | Teacher |

FIGURE 2.2 A representation of the relationship within a collaboration model

EXAMPLE

The educational psychologist and teacher jointly set aims and plan a behaviour modification programme to be carried out and reviewed together at regular intervals. They share knowledge and ideas in a reciprocal relationship, wherein the educational psychologist includes the teacher's objectives into her work and vice versa.

In this way, the teacher may share examples of situations in the classroom that the young person is experiencing difficulties with and the educational psychologist may explain why these difficulties are occurring from a behavioural perspective. The teacher and educational psychologist can agree priorities, set functional targets and devise a programme that includes opportunities for planned teaching as well as ideas for generalisation into everyday situations.

The collaboration model is more effective in encouraging sharing of knowledge and skills and creating a more equal relationship. It also encourages more consistent reinforcement of emerging skills, as the team members develop a greater awareness of what, how and why they are working on specific skills. This works both ways, as the educational psychologist, for example, has a greater understanding of the context in which the behaviours occur (how often the behaviours happen, what triggers the behaviours and what are the consequences of the behaviours, etc) and the teacher develops a greater understanding of the underlying factors of why the behaviours occur and how to promote more positive behaviours across all contexts.

This model often works well, but there may be disadvantages to this way of working. At times, the relationship may be influenced by differences in personality. In these situations, it may be difficult to prioritise the needs of the young person above these differences in personality.

Often, individual professionals are employed by different services within an agency or indeed different agencies. Therefore, the focus of intervention and the methods of service delivery adopted may significantly differ or change depending, for example, on the priorities or financial position of the employer at any time. This can make establishing and maintaining a reciprocal relationship difficult, however enthusiastic the individual professionals may be.

In addition, the approach is not holistic and may only address issues within the remit of the individual professionals working together. Depending on the type and location of service delivery, the needs of parents and carers may not be taken into account. For example, the educational psychologist and teacher may be working on a behavioural programme within the school setting and therefore find it difficult to assess the needs of the young person at home and provide advice and support to the family.

The transdisciplinary model

The collaboration model may be a very effective model of service delivery in some situations. Over time, working closely together may lead to a transdisciplinary approach (Kashman & Mora, 2002), where professionals can assume each other's roles. In our experience, this has been the most successful approach and forms the framework for this book. The transdisciplinary approach is the ultimate goal when working in a team. It ensures that opportunities for learning and development for the young person are continuous and not reliant on specific people or contexts. Ideally, this transdisciplinary model should encompass the professional team, the young person and the young person's parents or carers.

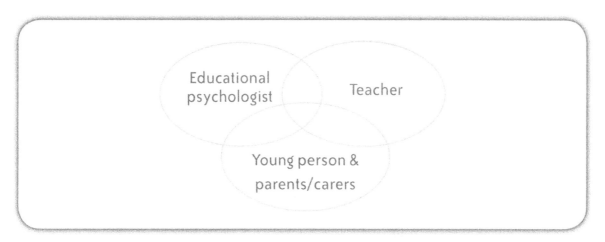

FIGURE 2.3 A representation of the relationship within a transdisciplinary model

EXAMPLE

The educational psychologist and teacher have learned skills and techniques from each other through sharing knowledge and experience and apply these independently across a range of contexts. They are able to assume each other's roles in similar situations that arise in the future (due to role release and expansion), whilst maintaining links that enable them to refer back to each other for further specialist advice where needs are different or more complex. The teacher, for example, has a clearer understanding of positive behaviour management strategies and is able to apply this knowledge to other young people in the classroom environment as needs are identified, whilst the educational psychologist has a better understanding of the demands of the curriculum and school environment and can tailor assessments and interventions more specifically towards meeting these challenges in the future. In addition, the educational psychologist and teacher liaise with parents and carers and the young person to share information and skills to ensure generalisation of skills into the home.

Transdisciplinary working involves the transfer of knowledge and skills between individuals in the team (including parents or carers and the young person) and requires a degree of trust between individuals that enables release (ie, sharing your knowledge and skills with others) and expansion (ie, acquiring new knowledge and skills from other professionals) of roles between team members. All of this leads towards the integrated approach we are advocating. This sharing of knowledge and skills and the process of role release and expansion can be developed through regular peer review sessions (see Chapter 6), during which reflection on the individual's and team members' performance can be encouraged. Discussion about how to improve the team members' performance and therefore enhance the young person's learning and potential for change can take place. This encourages a more holistic and integrated approach to education and intervention and is the foundation on which this book builds.

However, this is a challenging process and team members must feel confident and secure in their own and others' abilities. In our experience, this is a radical change in the usual way of working for many professionals and takes time to develop. Once established, though, the benefits are immense both to the young person and his family and to the professionals in the team.

The holistic and integrated approach to working with young people with ASD that the activities in this book provide lend themselves well to a transdisciplinary way of working. They should also be helpful to more recently established teams aiming to develop shared knowledge and skills and explore role release and expansion further.

Assessment

○ Why is assessment important?

Before planning a group, assessment of potential group members is required. This is important for a number of reasons. Firstly, it ensures that group members are matched appropriately by age and/or ability. Secondly, it helps to establish a profile of each young person's abilities and needs that will inform the general aims of the group. Finally, it enables the group facilitators to set targets for each group member against which to measure the outcomes of intervention.

○ Who carries out the assessment?

Each professional involved with the young person will usually complete an assessment from her own perspective. For example, an occupational therapist may look specifically at sensory issues and promoting independence in activities of daily living, whereas a speech & language therapist may focus on language development and socialisation. Professionals have a selection of formal standardised and informal observational assessment tools at their disposal.

○ Formal standardised assessment

These assessments show how a young person is performing in comparison with his peers. They can indicate delays and deviations from what is expected of a young person at a given age. An example of a comprehensive functional assessment that we have found useful is the Vineland Adaptive Behaviour Scales (Sparrow, 1984), which is carried out by the parent or carer and the young person themselves.

Formalised assessments usually assess a specific area of a young person's development (eg, expressive language, cognitive ability or fine motor skills). Few assessments give a concise overview of all of the areas that you may want to know about when planning a group. It is important to gather reports from all members of the team to build up a complete picture of the young person's strengths and needs. In addition, you are likely to require additional information that can be gathered through informal observational assessment.

○ Informal observational assessment

Informal assessments often catch the young person in a more natural setting (eg, at home or in the community) than can be achieved with formal assessment procedures. We have found informal assessments extremely useful in gathering the wide range of information we need to create a profile for a young person.

Informal assessment may include talking to the young person and/or his parents or carers, and observing him during a leisure or social activity or completing activities (eg, doing his homework, going shopping or making a hot drink).

Observing him across different settings and at different times of the day is desirable. Young people with ASD tend to use their skills variably in different situations. You may find, for example, that a young person can initiate conversation with his best friend at school but not with a group at lunchtimes, or that he is more sociable in the evenings without the demands of the school environment to worry about.

Informal observational assessments need to be focused and organised, as you need to know what you are looking for, how you will record the information, how long for and how you will use the information. With more able and mature young people, their opinions and views should be sought as you are more likely to get a young person involved in working towards change if they have identified the need and wish to do so. We have developed informal assessment profiles to use with parents and carers and the young person themselves that you may wish to use to supplement existing information and to assist you when planning a group. These can be found at the end of the chapter.

The information you gather from the team as well as the information gained from the supplementary assessment tools can be plotted onto an Assessment summary sheet and used to develop general group aims and the young people's targets.

○ Assessment guidelines

The checklists that we provide at the end of this chapter may be used alongside existing information gathered from other members of the team. These assessments can be used to gather the information that you will need in planning and preparing for the group to develop general group aims, set targets for the young people and review group progress.

Both the checklist to use with parent and carers and the one to carry out with the young person are designed to gather information about:

○ What is important to the young person and his parent/carer
○ How aware he is about his:
— Diagnosis
— Strengths and needs
— Functional skills of daily living
— Level of independence

Completing the assessment profiles

Parent/carer assessment profile

We would recommend completing the Parent/carer assessment profile first. This ensures that you have a good working knowledge of the young person and can provide the appropriate support when helping him to complete the Self-assessment profile. A minimum of one hour should be given to complete the profile with the parent or carer, but you may find you need longer than this, depending on the complexity of the young person's needs or the issues arising at any given time.

Self-assessment profile

This assessment is best completed with a group facilitator as some of the concepts and questions may cause young people difficulty. This also gives the facilitator an opportunity to develop an understanding of the young person's perceptions and understanding.

Both assessment profiles are designed to be carried out within an informal interview with a group facilitator, and could be completed within the pre-group meeting. This ensures that you get full and detailed information and provides the opportunity to explore any issues or concerns in greater depth. It also enables the group facilitators to get to know the young person and make an informed decision about the appropriateness of the group for him.

The assessment profiles should be signed by all of those completing the form. The forms and information should be copied with consent and shared with all relevant team members (including the young person and his parent or carer).

Assessment summary sheet

The Assessment summary sheet that we have provided is used to consolidate the information about the young person's strengths, needs and agreed targets. We suggest that you work with the young person and their parent or carer to identify three key areas that they would like to work on within the group. Plot these onto the table as agreed targets to be reviewed after every group session. For example, you may choose to focus on improving telephone skills, improving self-confidence and initiating conversation with others. There may also be issues that require referral to other agencies, for example, concerns about anxiety or depression would be referred to a child and adolescent mental health service at this point.

Parent/carer assessment profile

NAME OF YOUNG PERSON [ ]   DATE OF BIRTH [ ]

ASSESSED BY [ ]   DATE OF ASSESSMENT [ ]

INFORMATION PROVIDED BY [ ]

RELATION TO THE YOUNG PERSON [ ]

SECTION A: The young person's perceptions about diagnosis, strengths and needs

Diagnosis

Please specify the young person's diagnosis.

What does the young person know about this diagnosis?	
What does the young person feel they do well?	
What would the young person like to do better?	

SECTION B: The parent's/carer's perceptions about the young person's developmental skills

LANGUAGE AND COMMUNICATION SKILLS	
Understanding of verbal communication (literal interpretation, sarcasm, humour, following instructions)	
Understanding of non-verbal communication (understanding facial expressions, tone of voice, body language)	

Routledge
Taylor & Francis Group
ROUTLEDGE

Use of expressive language (using concise, clear sentences, keeping on topic)	
Ability to use non-verbal communication (eye contact, facial expression, gesture)	

IMAGINATION

Any difficulties in abstract thinking (time, empathy, insight)	
Routines (dislikes breaks in school or changes to home life)	
Obsessions or compulsions (gets stuck on one specific topic, needs to do things in the same way)	
Special interests (interest beyond what would be acceptable in other young people, such as bus routes, electrical wiring)	

SOCIALISATION

Motivation to engage with others (wants to join in with peers)	

Ability to initiate interactions [asks to join in, asks for help]	
Ability to maintain conversation [asks relevant questions, expresses interest in what others have to say]	
Social responses [responds to 'small talk']	
Social understanding [awareness of the need to modify behaviour in different situations]	
Friendships [How easy is it for them to make and maintain friendships? Do they understand what a friendship is about?]	
Girlfriend/boyfriend [Do they have one, want one or think they will meet someone in the future?]	
SENSORY SKILLS	
Are there any areas where the young person appears oversensitive or tries to avoid certain situations due to sensory issues? [does not like loud noises, the feel of labels in clothing]	

Routledge Taylor & Francis Group

Are there any areas where the young person seeks sensory input or struggles to process this? (seeks lots of movement or touch)	

MOTOR SKILLS

Fine motor skills (handwriting, computer skills)	
Gross motor skills (ball games, running, balance)	

COGNITIVE SKILLS

Attention and concentration	
Organisation and planning	
Memory	
Problem-solving	

EMOTIONAL ISSUES

Mood (fluctuation of moods, extremes of mood)	
Temper (loses temper easily)	

Routledge
Taylor & Francis Group
ROUTLEDGE

Self-esteem (is a confident person/lacks confidence/is happy with themselves)	
Anxiety (becomes anxious easily, displays no anxieties)	

DAILY LIVING SKILLS

Dressing (interest in fashion, predicting weather, matching clothes)	
Meal times (food preferences)	
Hygiene (awareness of need to shower, interest in personal hygiene)	
Meal preparation (prepares snacks, drinks, whole meals)	

COMMUNITY SKILLS

Groups/clubs they attend	
Ability to use public transport	

Groupwork for Children with ASD Ages 11–16 © A Eggett, K Old, LA Davidson & C Howe 2008

Routledge
Taylor & Francis Group
ROUTLEDGE

Money management	
Road safety	
Community independence skills (using the telephone, going to a restaurant)	

BEHAVIOUR

Behaviours observed (aggression, confrontation, passivity, withdrawal)	

COPING STRATEGIES

Coping strategies used (isolation, retreat to obsessions, talking to others, listening to music, using the internet)	

ANY OTHER ISSUES

SIGNED – GROUP FACILITATOR

SIGNED – PARENT/CARER

Routledge
Taylor & Francis Group

Self-assessment profile

This assessment is best completed by the young person and the group facilitator together.

NAME

DATE OF BIRTH   DATE OF ASSESSMENT

PROFESSIONAL PRESENT

SECTION A: General overview	
What diagnosis have you been given?	
What do you think this means?	
What do you do well? What do you think are your strengths?	
What would you like to do better? (eg, making friends, school work)	
What activities do you like to do? Why do you like these?	
Are there any activities you really don't like? Why don't you like these?	

SECTION B: Detailed information	

LANGUAGE AND COMMUNICATION SKILLS

This section deals with how well you think you communicate in different ways, with different people and in different situations.

Verbal communication How well do you understand what people say? (Are you able to follow instructions, understand jokes and know when things are not meant to be taken literally?)	

Routledge Taylor & Francis Group

How well do you think you express yourself? (Can you always say what you want? Do you always use clear sentences? Do you get distracted easily?)	
Non-verbal communication How well can you use non-verbal communication? (eye contact, facial expression, gesture)	
How well do you understand non-verbal communication? (how people use facial expression, eye contact and body position to communicate or add to what they say)	

IMAGINATION

This section deals with issues related to how flexible your thinking and behaviour are.

Do you have any difficulties in abstract thinking? (time, understanding others' point of view, empathy and insight, etc)	
How do you feel about breaks in routine: a) at home? b) at school?	
Do you have any obsessions or compulsions? (needing to do things in the same way, getting stuck on one specific topic)	

Routledge
Taylor & Francis Group

| Do you have any special interests? (unusual interests or interest beyond what would be seen in other young people, such as bus routes, electrical wiring, computers) | |

SOCIALISATION

This section deals with how well you manage social situations.

| How important is it for you to interact with other people? | |

| Do you have any problems with starting up a conversation? (asking to join in, asking for help) | |

| How do you think you manage with responding to social interactions? (Can you ask relevant questions? Can you express interest in what others have to say?) | |

| Do you have any difficulties in understanding social situations? (Do you understand the need to behave differently in different situations and the differences in relationships such as friend/teacher?) | |

| What about friendships? Do you find it easy to make friends? Do you have a close friend? | |

P This page may be photocopied for instructional use only. *Groupwork for Children with ASD Ages 11–16* © A Eggett, K Old, LA Davidson & C Howe 2008

Routledge
Taylor & Francis Group
ROUTLEDGE

Do you have a boyfriend/girlfriend? Would you like one?	

SENSORY SKILLS

This section deals with how you process and respond to sensory information such as noise, touch and movement.

Are there any sensory experiences that make you feel oversensitive and/or are keen to avoid? (loud noises, the feel of labels in clothing, certain tastes or movements)	
Are there any sensory experiences that you like? (lots of movement or touch, etc)	

MOTOR SKILLS

This section looks at how co-ordinated you are.

Do you have any problems with your fine motor skills? (handwriting, computer skills)	
Do you have any problems with your gross motor skills? (ball games, running, team sports)	

COGNITIVE SKILLS

This section deals with your thinking skills.

Do you have any problems with attention and concentration?	

Routledge
Taylor & Francis Group
ROUTLEDGE

Do you have any problems with organisation and planning?	
How well do you remember things?	
How good are you at problem-solving?	

EMOTIONAL ISSUES

This section deals with how you are feeling and how this affects how you think about yourself.

How would you describe your mood in general? (Do you have mood swings? Are you generally happy or fed up?)	
Do you have any problems with your temper?	
How would you describe yourself? (Are you a confident person or do you lack confidence? Are you happy with yourself?)	
Do you have any problems with anxiety? What do you get anxious about?	

Routledge
Taylor & Francis Group

DAILY LIVING SKILLS

This section deals with how you manage activities that you do every day.

Do you have any problems with dressing? (not being able to do fasteners, not being able to match clothes to weather conditions, choosing clothes for different occasions)	
Do you have any problems at meal times? (Do you only like a few things to eat? Can you prepare snacks and drinks without help from others?)	
Can you manage your own personal hygiene? (Do you know when to shower? Does anyone ever comment on your hygiene?)	

COMMUNITY SKILLS

This section looks at how you manage within the community.

Do you attend any groups/clubs?	
How do you find using public transport?	
Do you manage your own money?	

Do you feel you have good traffic awareness and road safety?

ANY OTHER ISSUES

SIGNED
(young person)

IN THE PRESENCE OF
(group facilitator)

Assessment summary sheet

NAME

DATE OF BIRTH   **DATE OF COMPLETION**

COMPLETED BY

SUMMARY OF STRENGTHS

IDENTIFIED NEEDS

AGREED TARGETS (to be reviewed after every session)

1

2

3

GROUP FACILITATOR'S SIGNATURE

PARENT'S/CARER'S SIGNATURE

GROUP MEMBER'S SIGNATURE

Routledge
Taylor & Francis Group

Planning a group

4

The benefits of groupwork

We have found groupwork to be a successful therapeutic treatment approach for young people with ASD. It provides a safe and structured environment in which to develop, practise and transfer the skills that young people with a diagnosis of ASD can find difficult.

In order to maximise learning opportunities, we feel it is beneficial to begin groupwork at an early stage of development, such as the early school years, and to continue this into adolescence, changing the group aims as the needs of the group members alter. For example, in the early years, the focus may be on establishing an effective communication system within a play situation, whereas by adolescence the focus is on using this system functionally within activities of daily living such as shopping. The groups are designed to develop the needs of every group member within each activity. The success of the activity is reviewed and altered as appropriate.

In our view, groupwork for older children and adolescents provides an opportunity for developing the following skills:

- Language and communication
- Socialisation
- Leisure time
- Sensory issues
- Motor skills
- Behaviour
- Emotional development
- Understanding of diagnosis
- Transitions
- Self-awareness and coping strategies
- Independent living skills

Our approach is intended to be functional and to teach skills in situ, thereby emphasising and encouraging the generalisation of skills into everyday, real-life situations. For example, the group members may explore tastes during Knowing your preferences (Activity 11) within the group setting with the ultimate aim of raising their awareness of their sensory preferences and developing coping strategies within a restaurant. A team approach facilitates generalisation, as all those involved with the young person (including the individual themselves) develop shared goals and aim to adopt consistent approaches that can be used outside the group setting.

○ Selecting the group members

We have found it best to group young people according to their age, for example, 11–13 years (emerging independence) and 14–16 years (facilitating independence).

At the *emerging independence* stage, group members are developing skills and beginning to generalise these into everyday situations with high levels of direction and support.

At the *facilitating independence* stage, the group members are using skills more autonomously by planning, preparing and carrying out activities with decreasing levels of direction and support.

Selecting group members in this way allows for appropriate selection of materials, equipment, activities and locations for community visits. All group members share recognised difficulties in a range of developmental areas, which impact on their activities of daily living, relationships, self-awareness, self-esteem, behaviour and social interaction and their ability to cope with transitions. It is important to allow for a degree of skill mix amongst the group members to encourage and enable the modelling of appropriate behaviour and communication to occur.

For these groups, we feel it is important to ensure that the age bands are adhered to because of differences of interests and issues relating to particular life stages (eg, transition from secondary school to further education or issues about having girlfriends/boyfriends). As with other groupwork programmes at different age bands, we continue to encourage mixed-sex groups; however, group facilitators may find that in some situations it is more appropriate to group all males or all females together to complete some activities or discuss certain topics (eg, relationships, puberty or sexuality).

The Group referral form (Appendix I) has been designed to help in the recruitment and selection of members for the group. We have found it useful to promote the group with the team of professionals and parents and carers to ensure appropriate referrals are made and plenty of candidates are available.

○ The size of the group

We have found that six is the ideal number of group members, as this allows for a good mix of skills, personalities and experiences but still allows opportunity for everyone to have a turn and for targets to be achievable within the time frame of the group. Four is the minimum recommended number, as any less than this makes the above very difficult to achieve.

A minimum of two group facilitators is essential. Any more depends on the individual needs of the group members, group dynamics and the group general aims. A higher ratio may be necessary if the group is going on community visits or is considered a high risk in terms of some of its members. Be aware, however, that too many group facilitators can impact on group dynamics and hinder opportunities to move towards independence.

○ The aims of the group

Pre-planned groups are not always effective as issues can arise during the course of the group (eg, exclusion from school, bereavement or bullying). We have found it useful to set general group aims, but to plan flexibly and review individual targets on a weekly basis. Each session should be loosely planned in advance by the group facilitators but the plan should be discussed in the group at the start of the session and agreed or modified according to any issues raised by the group members. This is particularly pertinent at the facilitating independence stage, where group members are encouraged to be more independent and take responsibility for identifying their own needs and targets. As a result, the Session plan sheet for the facilitating independence stage (Appendix IV) is set out slightly differently to encourage more flexibility.

The Session plan sheet should be displayed prominently in the group room for all group members and group facilitators to refer to. This may serve as a visual timetable itself, or the information may be needed to be transferred onto a visual timetable in a different format (see Chapter 5) for some group members. In the 11–16 age group, it is anticipated that group members will be working closer together as a team and forming a more cohesive unit so a shared session plan or timetable is used to encourage and support this. In comparison, pre-school (3–5) and primary school (5–11) children attending groups may still require individual resources to be provided as they learn to share and co-operate with their peers.

During a group session, we had agreed to carry out a community visit to the shops. The group facilitators had planned to use role plays (Activity 31) on buying items from a shop in preparation. One group member, **OMAR**, arrived quiet and withdrawn for this session. This was observed by the group facilitators, who responded by introducing the activity Good and bad things from the week (Activity 28). During this, Omar shared a bad experience he had gone through with another pupil at his school that day. The group facilitators therefore altered the focus of the session to explore Omar's and other group members' experiences of bullying. They encouraged discussion of this issue, getting group members to problem-solve the situation and to identify coping strategies. The next week, the group repeated Good and bad things from the week to give Omar a chance to discuss how things had gone and to assess the need for further group activities about bullying. By allowing this flexibility, the group members were able to resolve the issues around bullying and, by mutual agreement, the shopping trip was postponed to a later date. Giving the group members ownership of the sessions in this way promoted their confidence and strengthened the relationship with the group facilitators.

Preparing for a group

Holding a pre-group meeting

Before the group begins, a one-to-one session is carried out with each prospective group member and his parent or carer. For some group members, it may be appropriate to hold a separate meeting from their parent or carer. For example, practical reasons such as work or school commitments may prevent the young person and the parent or carer attending together or it could be that the parents and carers may wish to discuss sensitive issues that it would not be appropriate for the group member to hear, such as if family conflict or confrontations may be expected.

This meeting is to outline the general group aims and to provide information regarding the session times, venue and potential activities. The group member and his parent or carer are invited to share their feelings with regards to joining a group and to identify targets of their own, for example, using the telephone or using the bus independently. It is always the decision of the family whether they decide to attend the group.

Ideally, all group members will have met at least one of the group facilitators prior to the group commencing. This ensures an appropriate skill mix has been identified for the group and also helps to reduce anxieties about joining the group as the young person is familiar with at least one person who will be there. We often find that we have more success in achieving a group member's targets and that the group is a more positive experience for him when he has an established rapport with at least one of the group facilitators. If this is the first time the young person has been invited to a group, he may be offered some further individual or paired sessions in preparation.

The pre-group meeting allows for consent to be sought for community visits, photographs and videos (see Appendix II for a consent form). It also enables the group facilitator to gather information on specific health or dietary requirements, for example, if a young person needs a gluten- or casein-free diet and whether he is taking any medication.

Deciding on the venue and location

The group venue is selected according to the age and specific needs of the group. For example, a clinic-based environment may be more appropriate at the emerging independence stage, as the focus is less on community visits and more on developing skills that need to be learned in a safe environment. Smaller meeting-style rooms are more suited to the facilitating independence stage as the groups are focused on group members learning about themselves and their diagnosis, and more time is spent out on community visits (see Chapter 8).

At the emerging independence stage, the rooms should be big enough to be divided into different areas or zones. This helps to minimise distractions and to improve attention and concentration in the group. Ideally, we set up the following areas:

- Sensory and chill-out zone
- Motor activities area – including space for an obstacle course
- Table/floor space – this is useful for completing activities and snack time

Other considerations are listed in Table 4.1.

Over the years, we have found it impossible to find the ideal group venue. We have often had to borrow space in a variety of settings (eg, community centres and schools), all of which have had their disadvantages. We have had to be creative, using careful planning and portable equipment, and adapting the activities to the space available. A poor venue has even been used as a topic for the group members to discuss and provided them with problem-solving opportunities. At all times, we have had to place safety as our top priority and ensure that appropriate risk assessments are in place.

ESSENTIAL	DESIRABLE
Consider how the room is decorated, eg, remove distractions or create a more stimulating environment, depending on the needs of the group members. Be aware of age-appropriate décor as clinics can often cater more for babies and toddlers, and this can be viewed negatively by teenagers.	Lockable cupboard/storage space for large equipment, eg, trampoline, therapy ball and scooter board.
	Parking facilities.
Ensure that you have selected a safe environment that has no direct access by the general public. It should also have lockable windows and doors that can be shut, and easy access to toilet facilities.	Close proximity to public transport.
	Access or space to soft play/gym equipment/chill out area.
Ensure that the room provides privacy and confidentiality – it is useful to put up a sign indicating that the room is in use, which will help to avoid any interruptions.	Facilities for practising independent living skills, eg, making hot drinks, preparing snacks and telephoning.

TABLE 4.1 Essential and desirable considerations for the venue

At the emerging independence stage, we have found it very useful to provide a quiet area with tea and coffee facilities for the parents and carers. Many have commented on the positive benefits of meeting other families and sharing their experiences. On occasions, and with the consultation of parents and carers, outside speakers have been arranged to run parallel to the group; for example, a speaker from the local social services department might attend to discuss the services and benefits available to the families.

Crèche facilities are an added bonus where parents and carers have siblings to take care of. We have found that, at the facilitating independence stage, it has become more common for young people to access the group independently, being dropped off by their parent or carer or by school transport. However, when a group has been long established, the parents and carers may still choose to meet during group times and it is useful to have a room available for this.

It is important to consult the families when organising the venue, dates and times for the group, as in our experience this helps to increase attendance rates.

At both emerging and facilitating independence stages, the emphasis is on transferring and generalising the skills learnt in the clinic-based environment into the community setting. This has to be well-planned and with the consultation and consent of parents and carers. It is essential that a thorough risk assessment of the individual activity and each group member is carried out prior to any community visit. (Refer to your local risk assessment policies and procedures.)

When going on community outings at the emerging independence stage, parents and carers should try and bring the young person to the session and take them home afterwards. The eventual aim is to reduce this level of parent/carer involvement. This leads to independent access to groups for young people at the facilitating independence stage. This can take the form of using public transport or walking to the venue, depending on the activity itself, the time available, the ability of the group member and having parental consent.

CASE STUDIES

AIDAN is 14 years old, attends mainstream school and has used the bus independently to go to school for two years. It was agreed with Aidan, his parents and the group facilitators that he would get the bus to the group by himself. LIAM is also 14. He attends a different mainstream school but is on the same bus route as Aidan. Liam is not using public transport independently.

Aidan and Liam realised that they lived in the same area and shared the same bus route. They told the group facilitators that they would like to get the bus together to the group. With careful planning and negotiation with Aidan and Liam, their parents and group facilitators, it was agreed that Liam would begin to access the same bus route as Aidan.

The group facilitators were able to support this target in the group by carrying out Role plays (Activity 31) and Thought showers (Activity 33) in preparation for using public transport (Community visit F).

The timing of the group

When planning groups, it is important to consider the academic and social commitments of the group members. For example, exam time is best avoided, and summer often clashes with family holidays and clubs. The start of the academic year may be especially stressful for some young people and the group may be too much for them to deal with at that time. It is important to consider the individual make-up of the group, as some may benefit from the support at stressful times, such as exams, or during transitions.

○ What to do when the group is not working for a young person

Despite all the careful planning and preparation, it can become clear that it is not the right time for a young person to attend groupwork. There may be a number of reasons for this and we have identified some of the factors that we have found can contribute:

- Social issues may be causing difficulty settling in the group (for example, family breakdown, or moving house)
- Severe challenging behaviours (which may be the result of social issues or medical/health/mental health problems)
- Increasing awareness of their ASD diagnosis and difficulty managing feelings related to this
- Inconsistency in approach or management of behaviours between parents/carers and professionals
- Medical/health reasons
- Competing appointments
- The young person lacking motivation or not engaging with groupwork

In these situations, peer review is extremely important in identifying problems and implementing change. First, we try to make the group work for the young person. If this is not realistic however, we endeavour to find an alternative, even if this is having a break from intervention.

Before making changes, it is essential to discuss with the family and the young person (this may need to be done separately) why the group is no longer appropriate at this stage and for an alternative to be offered, if desired and appropriate.

CASE STUDY

MADDISON is 12 years old. Her family have recently moved house and she has subsequently started a new school. Maddison has regularly attended groupwork sessions with both group facilitators since the age of 9; she is also familiar with some of the group members from previous groups she has attended.

By Session 3, it was becoming clear that Maddison was finding the group difficult and not coping with the content of the sessions. She was becoming increasingly challenging by shouting out, disrupting others' work and requesting to go home. This was in direct contrast to her behaviour in other groups.

Following peer review, it was agreed that a meeting should be called with Maddison's mum and dad to share our concerns regarding her difficult presentation in the group. The meeting revealed that, after an initial settled period, she was now finding it difficult to cope in her new home and school, and similar behaviours had been noted in both settings.

The group facilitators discussed this with Maddison, who was clearly finding it difficult to express her feelings about the recent changes in her life. It was suggested that she may need some time away from the group so that she could be given some space to adjust to these changes. Onward referral was made to the local child psychology service and the school was kept informed of the situation as she accessed individual sessions with the psychologist. Once it became clear that the issues had been resolved, Maddison rejoined groupwork at a later date.

Running a group

Once the group members have been identified and general group aims set, it is time to begin looking at the practicalities of running the group. We have divided the groups by age into two stages:

Stage 1 (11–13 years) is referred to as *emerging independence*.
Young people working at the emerging independence stage need to develop prerequisite skills with higher levels of adult support.

Stage 2 (14–16 years) is referred to as *facilitating independence*.
Young people working at the facilitating independence stage will have acquired many of the prerequisite skills and will be working on generalising these into a functional community setting with graded levels of support.

Allowing time to plan

We have found it essential to set aside planning time in addition to the actual time allocated for running the group sessions. The amount of planning time that you need will depend on:

- The experience of the group facilitators
- Their familiarity with the other group facilitators
- Their familiarity with the group members
- The complexity of the group members' needs
- The suitability of the venue and any need for environmental adaptations

Planning time is often difficult to set aside. Most group facilitators will have additional responsibilities and other commitments alongside running the group. However, to ensure that the group runs effectively and successfully, try not to underestimate how much planning and preparation is required. Allow time to make lists of equipment and gather any photocopied worksheets. At least 30 minutes should be dedicated to this from the outset, but this time commitment may be reduced as you become more familiar with the activities and group members.

Make time just before each session to get the room ready, check equipment and set everything up. We recommend 15–30 minutes for this.

Planning group sessions

In our experience, it does not work to plan all the sessions from the outset. The group is designed to be flexible and respond to the needs of the group members, which can alter from session to session. This allows you to change activities in response to the group's performance and needs. During the session, you may find one activity is too difficult or too easy for a group, and that you need to alter the level or swap it for something else entirely. Alternatively, a group member may bring something they wish to discuss that alters the session plan.

The emerging independence stage

For emerging independence, a Session plan sheet is provided (Appendix III) to help you with choosing the activities. The form is designed to be used flexibly. For example, some groups may only require four activities alongside the warm-up activity, snack time and round-up activity, whereas others may need all six activities. There is also space to list the general aims for each session, the equipment or resources needed and to note down any comments following on from peer review.

The facilitating independence stage

Activities at the facilitating independence stage are designed to promote autonomy for the group, with the opportunity to plan, negotiate and influence group content. This must be done with the facilitators' support (see Chapter 4). Choose activities to aid this process, for example, Debates (Activity 30) or Thought showers (Activity 33).

Sessions can be easily adapted to meet group members' needs. For example, a group member may voice his concerns over upcoming exams and you may notice that he is becoming increasingly anxious. In this case, we would alter the session plan to include a thought shower on exam preparation and coping strategies.

The Group timetable (see Appendix V for an eight-week timetable, Appendix VI for an eighteen-week timetable) provides an overview of all of the sessions, for example, planned community outings or graded activities to develop ASD awareness. Individual Session plans (Appendix IV) can be created for each individual session in relation to this.

The duration and timing of the group

How long should the sessions last?

Sessions should last for 75–90 minutes, depending on the independence stage and group aims. Groups are held on an after-school basis wherever possible, allowing time for group members to travel to the venue.

How many sessions should there be?

At the facilitating independence stage, the number of sessions is determined by the aims of the group. For example, a group focusing on ASD awareness may run for eight sessions, whereas a group aiming to promote independent living skills in the community may run for twelve to eighteen sessions. We have found it beneficial to use natural breaks, such as school holidays, in the longer-running groups. This allows for consolidation and generalisation of skills learnt in the group into everyday settings. The template timetables (Appendices V and VI) can be adapted to suit the length and structure of your group sessions.

○ Choosing activities for a session

Structuring the session

When planning a session, we have found it helpful to maintain the same structure on a session-by-session basis, becoming more flexible at the facilitating independence stage. This is because the majority of individuals with ASD respond positively if a clear structure is in place. Our activities lend themselves to this approach by allowing for the different skill levels of group members. For example, an obstacle course can be done at the same time in each session. As the group gain confidence and skills with this activity, it can be made more challenging by moving onto the next level described in the activity.

Beginning and ending the session

We have found a consistent warm-up and round-up activity useful to define the beginning and end of the session. Parachute games (Activity 1) is especially useful for this at the emerging independence stage as it allows for a range of skills to be learned, increases group members' self-confidence and creates a sense of ease. However, you could pick any activity, as long as it is consistently done at the session beginning/end.

At the facilitating independence stage, during clinic-based sessions, we have found that it has been useful for group members to get a drink and snack as they arrive at the group. This helps to create a sense of ease within the group and promotes social chat. The mix of clinic and community sessions at this stage can make it difficult to maintain a consistent warm-up and round-up activity. However, the age and maturity of the group members at this stage make it more likely they will be able to cope with less consistency in the sessions.

For both levels, you need to be aware of the calming and alerting qualities of activities and consider each group member's sensory profile. You may need to introduce a calming or alerting activity into the session as appropriate. For example, group members may arrive at the group in a high state of excitability and may need a calming activity before they are able to concentrate on what you have planned. Again, this highlights why flexibility within each session is important. Do not be afraid to change activities according to the needs of the group at the time.

The first session

At the facilitating independence stage, we have found it useful to use the first group session to allow group members to negotiate and compromise on group content. We have provided a number of possible activities related to the group aims and the group members are encouraged to plot these across a session timetable (Appendix V or VI). For example, in a twelve-week session group, four or five community outings may be selected by the group members. These would then be plotted onto the timetable, allowing time for clinic-based sessions related to preparing for the outings. This means that an outing in the community needs to have a session before for preparation and a session after for debriefing. See the second working example at the end of Chapter 6 for an example of this.

Snack time

For the emerging independence stage, snack time is usually best at the midway point of the session. For the facilitating independence stage, snack time comes at the beginning of the session whilst the group members chat and plan the group session between them (eg, group members have a cup of tea/coffee whilst planning takes place). Physical activities, for example, obstacle courses, relays and circuits should be carried out before snack time.

○ General tips for the activities

At the emerging independence stage, some group members may find it difficult to stay in their position when seated on the floor. Some may need a round spot cut from paper or made from rubber to sit on. This creates a visual and tactile reminder to keep within their own space. The young people are encouraged to position themselves in order to promote self-regulation and eventually remove the need for a physical prompt.

Reduce or increase verbal and visual prompts according to each group member's needs. For example, one group member may need forced alternatives (eg, a choice of two options) to make choices, whereas another may not need any.

- Dissuade group members from shouting out and interrupting others. Discuss why this behaviour is not appropriate and give good models, or invite suggestions from other group members.

- Always explain the reasoning behind what you do and discuss this with the group. Young people with ASD may apply skills and ideas better if they have a firm understanding and opportunities to practise in real-life situations. For example, when teaching about personal space, you would discuss the situations where this would be important and why, before carrying out activities to explore this (eg, queuing in a shop).

- Modelling is a useful way of demonstrating all activities.

- A collage box (Appendix VII) is an excellent tool. Be on the lookout for things to add to it. When using the contents of the collage box, put it in the middle of the group to encourage turn-taking/sharing. Try to limit essential items (eg, one pair of scissors/glue pot for every three group members). This will encourage group members to have to ask each other for things. Be aware that some may need more support with this. Be prepared to identify inappropriate behaviour; say what is more appropriate and why. You may have to allow some young people to copy you asking in an appropriate way to begin with.

- For craft activities, it is worth thinking about using aprons to protect the group members' clothing and mats to cover the floor.

- When videoing or photographing activities a consent form (Appendix II) needs to be filled in by the parent/carer.

- Consider allergies and food sensitivities – a record of these should be added to the consent form (Appendix II) by the parent or carer.

Using visual timetables

At the emerging independence stage, we have found that a visual timetable is a useful method of reducing group members' anxiety with regards to what is coming next in the session. We designed a simple timetable using cardboard backing with a 'pocket' at the end. Symbols were then attached to the cardboard with a sticky strip

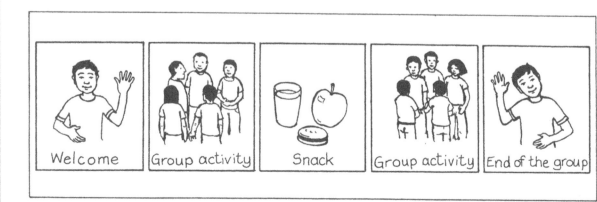

| Welcome | Group activity | Snack | Group activity | End of the group |

in chronological order. Symbols can be photographs, simple line drawings, a symbol from a published computer package and/or a written word, depending on the needs and abilities of the group. For the facilitating independence stage, a written list of activities can be provided if necessary.

Ensure that the visual and written timetables are as flexible as possible. We would recommend terms such as 'Welcome', 'Group activity 1' and 'Snack', rather than specifics such as 'Parachute games', 'Obstacle course' or 'Who am I?'. This allows for flexibility within the session, but still allows a structure to reduce any anxieties for group members about what is happening next.

Welcome
Group activity 1
Group activity 2
Snack
Group activity 3
Group activity 4
End of group

Emerging independence

At this stage, we have found it useful for one group member to have the role of timetable monitor. This means that they are responsible for removing the appropriate symbol from the timetable once that activity has finished. This allows for a degree of responsibility and promotes self-confidence for that group member.

Facilitating independence

At this stage, the group members can be encouraged to plan aspects of the session themselves and therefore should be encouraged to design, maintain and manage their own timetable. This can be negotiated within the group as to individual versus group timetables and a 'chair' can ensure that timetables are being adhered to.

Snack time

This is one of the most important aspects of the session. It is used to promote socialisation skills, such as turn-taking and listening. It provides time for exploring tastes and textures. It also introduces independent living skills, such as making juice (or tea and coffee at the facilitating independence stage) for themselves and their peers. Most importantly, it provides an opportunity for encouraging functional communication and generalisation of newly emerging skills that have been learned during other group activities.

In our experience, snack time is one of the most challenging times, both for group members and group facilitators, because of the high demand for unstructured social interaction. Once a routine is established, we have found snack time to be an excellent forum for developing a large range of skills, for example, initiating a conversation, keeping on topic or sequencing making a drink. Make targets small and manageable and do not try to target everything at once. For example, if your target is to get the young person to initiate conversation, do not place another demand on him such as tasting new foods.

Tips for running snack time

○ Ensure that there is enough room and space for group members to sit round the table for snack time.

○ Discourage wandering, but if sitting still for long periods is difficult, provide the group member with structured movement breaks, for example, take him to the kitchen to get paper towels or hand out snacks. At the facilitating independence stage, this can be used to promote self-regulation and to develop appropriate coping strategies.

○ Snack time provides an excellent opportunity for general chat and sharing of group members' news from the week. This is a skill that can take a while to develop; initially more structured conversations or use of worksheets (for example, see Appendices XIV–XVII) are a useful tool to help keep attention and group cohesion when social chat is challenging.

○ Provide a clear space for group members to make drinks. Allow for spillages, and have plenty of paper towels to hand. Be aware of health and safety concerns about making hot drinks and using electrical equipment.

○ Sometimes, you may wish the focus of this activity to be exploring different tastes and textures (eg, different flavoured crisps or different textured fruits). This is best done when the group is comfortable with the snack time routine.

The emerging independence stage

At this stage, select one group member to be the 'waiter' for each session, ensuring that each group member has a chance to try out this role. It is the waiter's responsibility to take group members' drink orders, make the drinks and hand them out. This often needs a high level of support from a group facilitator, with the aim being to gradually reduce this support. You will need to model asking group members what they would like to drink and them responding appropriately. You may need to get the waiter and the responding group member to copy what you say when it is their turn.

We have found that an 'order sheet' with group members' names down one side and space for marking their orders can help those group members who struggle to remember what others want. You may also consider using a visual sequence of how to make the drinks. This could be photographs or written instructions depending on the ability of the waiter.

It is also useful to nominate a different group member to hand out the snacks to the group while the drinks are being made. Again, ensure that this is being done appropriately and be prepared to model. Get group members to copy you if they are finding it difficult to ask appropriate questions or find appropriate answers. Ensure that the waiter is also offered a snack. This can lead to some lively discussions about social rules, for example, why you are meant to ask everyone else what they want before helping yourself.

The facilitating independence stage

At this stage, the emphasis shifts to group members making their own drinks and offering to make others a drink as they arrive at the session. Support will be needed to discuss issues about 'good manners' and thinking of others before themselves, linking this with their diagnosis as appropriate.

Initially, you may need to use models and prompts; however, these can be gradually reduced as the young person develops independence.

The use of video/DVD

Recording activities (eg, on video or DVD) is useful for giving feedback to young people, their parents/carers and the wider team. It also gives group members an opportunity to learn a new skill. For example, in Interviews (Activity 3), a young person may be encouraged to observe his non-verbal communication skills. This can increase self-awareness, and help to identify new targets and opportunities for change. It can also provide a less challenging role for those unsure of activities. A role behind the camera can reduce anxiety for these group members until they feel more confident to join in.

With consent, videos can also be used to train students and other professionals by giving examples of how to carry out group activities and by highlighting the characteristics of ASD and strategies that do or do not work with these young people.

Funding for community visits

Some of the community visits in Chapter 8 will require funding. We suggest that you refer to your local policies and management team to investigate sources of funding for such visits. You could involve your group in this. For example, during one group we got the group members to write their own letter to our management team outlining the outings they were planning, the aims of these outings and estimated costs. This helped the management team to understand the value of funding such community visits for this particular client group.

○ After a session

Once the group members have gone home, time must be allowed to debrief, keep records, complete peer reviews, consider observations and plan the next session (see Chapter 6).

○ After the group sessions have finished

Time needs to be set aside to produce group summary reports outlining the aims of the group, how each group member performed and recommendations for future groupwork (Appendix VIII). The time needed will depend on the experience of the group facilitators and the complexity of needs among the group members.

Consider offering individual appointments to parents, carers and/or the young people to feed back the contents of the report and discuss future management plans.

Give evaluation forms to group members and parents or carers to help you evaluate and plan further groups. We have developed separate Group member evaluation forms for emerging and facilitating independence stages (Appendices IX, X and XI). These can be given out at the end of the group to be returned at the feedback session.

Keeping records

6

○ Why do we need to keep records?

It is essential to keep records as part of the groupwork process. Keeping records will facilitate future group planning. For example, it may highlight issues that suggest the need to identify a different venue or alter the structure of the group sessions in response to your own or the group members' needs.

Records will also help you to make informed decisions about the young person's future needs. When they move on to new services or settings, the records can move with them and assist in the transition between services. This prevents repetition from occurring and provides new team members with useful strategies from the start, rather than a period of 'getting to know the young person' and discovering for themselves what works and what does not.

Some young people may be starting secondary school or moving into further education and the records will help you to form an opinion about the choice of educational placement, career pathway or their support needs. These records will help to identify what should be the next step in terms of advice, support and input. This may be different for each young person and could include one-to-one work, more groupwork, support for the family or referrals to other appropriate services. The records will provide the evidence that you need to support your decisions.

○ What information is needed?

When planning your group, ensure that you build in time for preparation and for the paperwork, alongside the actual group sessions. The time needed depends on the experience of the group facilitators. We would recommend a minimum of one hour per group session.

The records should include:

- General information about the group, including aims, the number of members attending, venue, number and structure of sessions and any issues that arise (for example, poor parking facilities or lack of storage space).
- Specific information about each young person, including individual targets, progress made, persisting difficulties and any other observations (for example, identified behaviour modification strategies).

Much of this information is recorded throughout the planning stages and following the group sessions. For example, the Assessment profiles, Assessment summary sheet and Session record sheets that we have produced provide details about the young person's abilities and needs, progress made and any additional observations, for example, strategies that worked or did not work.

As ASD is recognised as a life-long developmental disorder, many young people have ongoing needs (see Chapter 1). For this reason, these records are essential in helping us to monitor progress over time and to continually modify our targets and expectations for each group member, in line with their changing needs. They are a permanent record of the young person's achievements and of the individualised approach that has been developed to help him become more independent.

○ Sharing information

The information gained should, with consent, be shared with the whole team and new team members so that all those working with the young person have a complete and up-to-date picture of his progress and areas of continuing need. A Group summary report (Appendix VIII) should be completed that includes information about:

- The aims of the group
- The individual group member's targets
- His attendance
- His progress
- Recommendations and future action

There are numerous ways to record a young person's progress and to monitor areas of continuing need.

○ Note-keeping

After each group session, notes should be written to record the activities that the young person has engaged in, his response to these activities, progress made and any issues that arose. Notes should be written as soon as possible after the session finishes, whilst still fresh in the memory. At this time, the group member's targets can be reviewed and any modifications made ready for the next group session. Session record sheets are provided (Appendices XII and XIII) to facilitate with this process.

○ Using photographs and videos

With parental consent (Appendix II), we usually take photographs during every group session. A video recording is also taken in the first, middle and last session to record changes in behaviour and progress.

The photographs can be used to create visual helpers, to provide a memento of the group for the young person and his family and, most importantly, can be evidence of increased socialisation within the group. During one group, we took a photograph in the first session that showed each group member engaged in his own activity and showing limited awareness of the people around him. In comparison, a photograph taken in the last session showed the group members focused on the same activity and sharing resources.

Similarly, videos can be used to show evidence of increased socialisation. We also use videos for coaching purposes. The recordings are a permanent record of a young person's response to different activities, strategies and techniques. We often use videos to support discussion with the young person and within the group about their performance and specific behaviours. Coping strategies and techniques (such as using appropriate openings to conversations) can be tried out, recorded and played back to analyse in more detail what worked and what did not.

◎ Undertaking peer review

Each group session should be followed by a peer review that allows the group facilitators to analyse the performance of the supporting adults within each activity and their impact on the young person.

Peer review involves analysing the group facilitators' actions and behaviour during activities and identifying the factors that may have helped to achieve positive results or led to difficult behaviours (eg, inappropriate use of language or lack of co-operation).

Issues to be considered may include, for example:

- Were the activities sufficiently well-organised and structured?
- Were opportunities given for the group member to take his turn?
- The level of direction provided by group facilitators – was enough autonomy given to the group?
- Have group members been sufficiently involved in planning sessions and setting targets?
- Did the group facilitators use appropriate language?
- Were visual supports used effectively?
- Were appropriate resources/equipment used?
- Have risk assessments been reviewed and explained to group members?

Our own behaviour, communication and interactive styles can significantly influence how a young person responds. Peer review enables us to identify how we need to adapt what we do.

Peer review also provides an opportunity to discuss the influence of environmental factors (eg, noise levels) and how these are affecting the group member's performance. A section to summarise the factors noted within the peer review is included on the

SUNNI is 15 years old. Although he presents himself as a very confident and articulate young man, his understanding of language is very literal and he tends to interpret things in a very concrete way. During a visit to a café, he became very distressed and found it increasingly difficult to cope during conversations. He then became isolated and withdrawn from the rest of the group. During peer review, it was identified that the group facilitator supporting Sunni was using a lot of humour and sarcasm within conversation, which Sunni was unable to understand. In the next session, the group facilitators were more aware of their use of language and ensured they explained any sarcasm or humour to Sunni. This resulted in a discussion with the group about asking for clarification if any of them did not understand a word or phrase. By including the group in this, the spotlight was taken off Sunni. This provided Sunni and the group with strategies to use when they found themselves in similar situations in future.

JACK is 11 years old. During an activity using the feely bag, he became tearful and anxious each time he took a turn. The group facilitator interpreted this as difficulty relating to taking turns. During peer review, it was recognised that his reluctance to take part was due to tactile sensitivity and that insisting that he took a turn was causing more distress. In future activities, the group facilitators considered Jack's sensory issues and gave him gradual exposure and opportunities for time out.

Session plan (Appendix III – the emerging independence stage, Appendix IV – the facilitating independence stage) and should be referred to when planning the next group session and writing the Group summary report (Appendix VIII).

Professionals need to feel comfortable with this style of reflective practice and to accept praise and criticism equally from colleagues, alongside advice and suggestions for improving working practices. The consensus amongst the professionals within our own team is that working relationships need to be well-established in order to use reflective practice effectively so that this leads to a positive cross-discipline learning experience that enables professionals to share their knowledge and the skill mix. In turn, this ensures that the group member is provided with the optimum learning environment to maximise progress and leads to a more transdisciplinary approach evolving (see Chapter 2).

Working example 1 planning & running a group for members at the emerging independence stage

This group was facilitated by an assistant psychologist with an interest in ASD and a specialist teacher from a unit for pupils with ASD. The group is made up of five pupils from the specialist unit. The individual profiles of the young people in the group are as follows.

XIAO XI is 13 years old. She was diagnosed with ASD last year and is only just beginning to accept this. She was transferred from mainstream education to the specialist unit three months ago. On the surface, Xiao Xi seems to be coping with the change; however, her parents have noted an increase in obsessional behaviours and her need for sameness. Xiao Xi is coping academically but appears reluctant to mix with her peers and has begun to voice feelings of not fitting in with her new class.

ANDRE is 12 years old, with a diagnosis of ASD. He has been in specialist education since the age of four, following his diagnosis. Since the transfer to the secondary unit, Andre has begun to join his mainstream peers in a number of lessons. Andre has found it difficult to manage social interactions with more socially aware peers. Incidents have been reported where Andre has perceived the other boys as laughing with him; however, an observer felt that this was more that the other boys were laughing at Andre. His parents and teachers are concerned by these reports and feel that the amount of contact with these boys should be minimal. Andre is very angry and feels that he is being excluded from his peers.

JOANNA is 12 years old. She was diagnosed with ASD when she was 7 years old. She moved into specialist education when transferring from primary to secondary school. Joanna's younger sister also has ASD. Her parents are very supportive of both children. Although she can discuss her diagnosis, it is felt that her understanding of this is limited. Joanna appears to have a lack of awareness of how she is perceived by her peers. She has no interest in fashion and follows her own interests (card collecting) without concern about how this is viewed by the other girls.

DANNY is 13 years old, with a diagnosis of ASD and motor co-ordination difficulties. Danny spends the majority of his time within a mainstream school and attends the unit for support sessions. He has a number of friends and has taken upon himself the role of the class clown. Teachers perceive him as cheeky and disorganised, leading to misunderstandings and occasional detentions. At home, Danny expressed confusion over these detentions as he cannot understand the reasons for them. Danny's mum complains that she never receives important letters from school as Danny always loses them.

ALISDAIR is 13, with significant mental health difficulties, including regular 'lows'. Alisdair received his diagnosis of ASD when he was 11, following lengthy assessments relating to mental health issues. Alisdair is a bright boy; however, he is not motivated to engage in school work or peer relationships. He finds paired and groupwork extremely difficult. As much of the work in school involves groupwork, his teachers are concerned that he is missing out on important areas of the curriculum and may fall behind.

The group facilitators held an informal meeting with each set of parents prior to the group starting. Here, they discussed the general aims of the group and completed the Parent/carer assessment profile (see Chapter 3) in order to identify any issues outside of the school setting. As the group facilitators were very familiar with the young people, they used existing assessments and knowledge of the group members rather than carrying out the Self-assessment profiles with the group members.

The group facilitators were able to use this information to discuss and evaluate each young person's suitability and readiness for the group, and pull together individual targets for the group members. These targets were transferred to an Assessment summary sheet (see Chapter 3). Below are the targets for each group member.

Xiao Xi's targets

Agreed targets (to be reviewed after every session)
1 To develop an understanding of ASD
2 To develop her awareness of how her diagnosis impacts on her
3 To promote positive peer interactions

Andre's targets

Agreed targets (to be reviewed after every session)
1 To develop his understanding of social situations
2 To develop his ability to interpret non-verbal communication
3 To promote effective expression of feelings

Joanna's targets

Agreed targets (to be reviewed after every session)
1 To promote her awareness of ASD and how this relates to her
2 To develop an understanding of the value in having shared interests with peers
3 To develop her awareness that others may have different thoughts and beliefs to her own

Danny's targets

Agreed targets (to be reviewed after every session)
1 To explore different styles of verbal communication
2 To develop strategies to assist Danny in analysing challenging situations
3 To develop organisational skills

Alisdair's targets

Agreed targets (to be reviewed after every session)
1 To provide opportunities to develop turn-taking skills
2 To explore and express a range of feelings
3 To develop positive peer interactions

The group facilitators met for approximately one hour before the start of the first group session to discuss possible activities and themes that would promote the group members' targets. These ideas were plotted onto an eight-week timetable (Appendix V).

Group timetable – eight weeks

LOCATION Riverdale Community Centre

DATE TIMETABLE COMPLETED 05.09.XX

GROUP FACILITATORS PRESENT Lisa Moore, assistant psychologist
James Peterson, specialist teacher

NAMES OF GROUPWORK PARTICIPANTS Xiao Xi, Andre, Joanna, Danny & Alisdair

Session number	Session focus
1	<u>Activities to get the group together</u> People bingo (Activity 2) for getting to know you Zoo (Activity 23) to promote a sense of fun
2	<u>Self-awareness</u> Life maps (Activity 37) Good and bad things from the week (Activity 28) Give out letter for Show and tell (Activity 4)
3	<u>Self-awareness/Awareness of ASD</u> Show and tell (Activity 4) Quizzes (Activity 32) with ASD theme
4	<u>Awareness of ASD and feelings about this</u> Friendship darts (Activity 6) with ASD theme Interviews (Activity 3) with ASD theme
5	<u>Sharing emotions and experiences</u> What's in my head? (Activity 40) Act out emotions (Activity 34)
6	<u>Carrying on themes from Session 5 on how to manage angry feelings</u> Role plays (Activity 31)
7	<u>Understanding others</u> Compliments (Activity 7) Who am I? (Activity 22)
8	<u>Recap</u> Salt jars (Activity 8) on theme of positive characteristics of group members

Each session lasted for one-and-a-half hours over eight consecutive weeks. The sessions took place after school in a local community centre, as this was felt to separate the group from the school setting where some group members were experiencing difficulties. The centre was chosen due to its central location and good access to public transport for all the group members attending. It had a large group room to meet in, as well as a smaller room for individual group members and the group facilitators to go to if sensitive issues arose or a period of 'time out' from the whole group was needed.

On the following page is an example session plan for Session 3. The group facilitators met straight after school for an hour before the session to plan the activities, set up the room and collect equipment.

All sessions follow the same basic structure:

- Warm-up activity
- 2–3 activities
- Snack time
- 2–3 activities
- Round-up activity

The group facilitators discussed how the activities could be adapted to meet the group members' targets. It also gave them an opportunity to discuss any possible safety issues and ensure that a risk assessment had been completed.

Session plan sheet –
emerging independence stage

DATE OF SESSION 19.09.XX   **LOCATION** Riverdale Community Centre

SESSION START TIME 16.30   **SESSION END TIME** 18.00

GROUP FACILITATORS Lisa Moore, assistant psychologist
James Peterson, specialist teacher

GENERAL AIMS OF THE SESSION Self-awareness & awareness of ASD
(session 3)

Warm-up activity Parachute games (Activity 1)	Estimated time 5 mins
Activity 1 Mimes (Activity 19)	Estimated time 10 mins
Activity 2 Relays (Activity 16). Complete with tasks not requiring equipment	Estimated time 15 mins
Activity 3 n/a	Estimated time n/a
Snack time Alisdair to make drinks, Danny to pass round snacks	Estimated time 15 mins
Activity 4 Show and tell (Activity 4)	Estimated time 20 mins
Activity 5 Quizzes (Activity 32)	Estimated time 20 mins
Activity 6 n/a	Estimated time n/a
Round-up activity Parachute games (Activity 1)	Estimated time 5 mins

Session plan sheet – emerging independence stage continued

COMMENTS (to be completed after peer review)

RESOURCES NEEDED

Parachute, mime cards, drinks, cups, snacks and quiz questions

After the session, the group facilitators met to discuss and record how it went. They discussed each group member in turn and recorded their observations about them during the session. These observations were recorded on the Session record sheet (Appendix XII) and used to review the group members' targets and alter them if necessary. We have provided a summary of the key points from the Session record sheets of each group member as well.

The group facilitators also carried out a peer review to analyse their own behaviour, communication and interactive styles to identify any factors that may have significantly influenced the group members' performance. This was recorded in the 'Comments' section on the Session plan and used to modify the group facilitators' approach as required. We have provided a summary of the key points raised during peer review for each group member where relevant to illustrate important issues.

Summary of Session record sheet for Xiao Xi

Xiao Xi arrived at the group in a mood and announced that she did not want to be there as she wanted to be out with her friends. She reluctantly joined in the warm-up activity and first two activities. During snack time, Xiao Xi isolated herself from the group and would only answer direct questions from the group facilitators.

At Show and tell (Activity 4), Xiao Xi had no object to discuss. She said that she had not brought anything in because she did not want to discuss personal things in the group. As the activity progressed, Xiao Xi became very negative and disrespectful of her fellow group members.

In the final activity, Xiao Xi became upset and left the room. She could not be persuaded to rejoin her peers.

This was an escalation of a pattern of behaviour for Xiao Xi, seen over the previous two sessions. The group facilitators felt that the group was not meeting Xiao Xi's needs and that a meeting with Xiao Xi and her parents should take place to discuss alternative forms of support. Her targets remained unchanged at this time, with a view to reviewing them following the meeting with Xiao Xi and her parents.

Summary of key points from peer review

Peer review relating to Xiao Xi focused on how her negativity was managed within the group. As Xiao Xi was relatively new to the facilitators, discussion took place as to how to identify when Xiao Xi's behaviour may escalate, triggers and which approaches may work better than others (eg, time out being more effective than encouragement).

Summary of Session record sheet for Andre

During the mimes (Activity 19), Andre positioned himself with his back to his peers, thus blocking their view. He became annoyed when asked to move to one side. Following the relay (Activity 16), Andre and Danny had a disagreement as Danny accused Andre of causing their team to lose. Andre could not acknowledge his part in this. During Show and tell (Activity 4), he talked in a mumbling voice and had to be prompted to speak up by his peers. This again resulted in Andre becoming upset and abandoning his show and tell. By the end of the session, Danny and Andre had made friends and won the quiz activity.

Andre's behaviour in the session indicates that his targets remain appropriate for the next session.

Summary of key points from peer review

Following peer review, it was suggested that in future sessions Andre would be paired with one of the other group members to promote more positive interactions. Andre was allocated a particular group facilitator to take him to one side when his angry feelings emerged to practise calming techniques and to discuss more effective ways of expressing his emotions.

Summary of Session record sheet for Joanna

Joanna enjoyed the parachute games (Activity 1) this week. She was very good at guessing other group members' mimes (Activity 19); however, when performing mimes she could not move away from her own special interests.

Joanna was very pleased to win the relays (Activity 16) and became overly excited, hugging Xiao Xi. She appeared unaware of Xiao Xi's reluctance to be hugged.

During the snack time, Joanna continued to try to bring the conversation around to her own interest. She appeared unaware of the verbal and non-verbal signals from other group members that they were losing interest in this topic of conversation.

Joanna participated fully in Show and tell (Activity 4), listening and making positive comments.

Joanna demonstrated good awareness of ASD in the quiz (Activity 32).

From Joanna's behaviour in this session and in particular her knowledge of ASD, it was decided that her targets should be changed as follows. These were added to the Assessment summary sheet and Session record sheet.

Joanna's revised targets

> **Agreed targets** (to be reviewed after every session)
> 1 To develop an understanding of how her ASD affects her relationships with others
> 2 To develop an understanding of the value in having shared interests with peers
> 3 To develop her awareness that others may have different thoughts and beliefs to her own

Summary of key points from peer review

Peer review in relation to Joanna focused on which approach proved most beneficial in helping her to realise her targets. During mimes, one group facilitator adopted a direct approach with Joanna, telling her that her fellow group members were bored with her repetitive themes as it made her mimes very easy to guess. The other group facilitator noted how well Joanna responded to this approach and it was decided that both should adopt this style with Joanna in future sessions.

Summary of Session record sheet for Danny

Danny found the parachute games (Activity 1) very difficult and tended to engage in silly behaviour. This set the tone for his approach for the rest of the session's activities.

During mimes (Activity 19), Danny was good at guessing and supportive of his peers. However, his mimes were very vague and difficult to guess and he was reluctant to take his turn or repeat any actions.

Danny became frustrated with Andre in the relays and teased him regarding his performance. This escalated and Danny struggled with how to manage this effectively. He was more settled when carrying out table-top activities and during snack time, where he handed out the snacks.

Following discussion of how the session went for Danny, the group facilitators decided to keep his targets the same.

Summary of key points from peer review

In peer review, discussion took place about the lack of opportunities to meet Danny's target regarding organisational skills. The group facilitators agreed to remedy this by putting him in charge of the visual timetable or getting him to organise a group obstacle course. It was also decided not to pair Danny with Andre in future competitive activities.

Summary of Session record sheet for Alisdair

Alisdair remained on the periphery of the group for the majority of the time; he tended to direct all conversation to group facilitators and was keen to opt out whenever possible. When given a role, Alisdair appeared to brighten and took more interest in the activity, for example when he was given the timer in the relay race (Activity 16).

In Show and tell (Activity 4), Alisdair was able to give a good presentation and accepted the group's comments.

Alisdair found the quiz (Activity 32) difficult and appeared to have a limited knowledge of ASD.

Following this session, Alisdair's targets were altered to include a target about awareness of ASD. These were amended on the Assessment summary sheet and Session record sheet.

Alisdair's revised targets

Agreed targets (to be reviewed after every session)

1 To provide opportunities to develop turn-taking skills
2 To explore and express a range of feelings
3 To develop positive peer interactions
4 To develop his knowledge of ASD

Summary of key points from peer review

In peer review, group facilitators discussed the need to give Alisdair shared tasks with another peer to develop peer interactions. It was also decided that the group facilitators should redirect conversation to include peers rather than adults.

Below is the plan for Session 4, outlining the planned activities and including details of things that the group facilitators needed to look out for following their observations and peer review of Session 3.

Session plan sheet – emerging independence stage

DATE OF SESSION 26.09.XX **LOCATION** Riverdale Community Centre

SESSION START TIME 16.30 **SESSION END TIME** 18.00

GROUP FACILITATORS Lisa Moore, assistant psychologist
James Peterson, specialist teacher

GENERAL AIMS OF THE SESSION Awareness of ASD and feelings about this (session 4)

	Estimated time
Warm-up activity Parachute games (Activity 1) Be aware of Danny becoming overstimulated	5 mins
Activity 1 Friendship darts (Activity 6) with ASD theme	15 mins
Activity 2 Obstacle course (Activity 15) Danny to design – give him some equipment to use Be aware of Danny and Joanna becoming overstimulated	20 mins
Activity 3 n/a	n/a
Snack time Alisdair and Joanna to agree on jobs	15 mins
Activity 4 Interviews (Activity 3) with ASD theme One-to-one support for Alisdair; pair Andre and Alisdair	20 mins
Activity 5 Zoo (Activity 23)	10 mins
Activity 6 n/a	n/a
Round-up activity Parachute games (Activity 1)	5 mins

Session plan sheet –
emerging independence stage

COMMENTS (to be completed after peer review)

RESOURCES NEEDED

Parachute, dart board, tunnel, hoop and ball for obstacle course, drinks, cups and snack, interview sheets – blank

The same process of reflection and modification of targets and the session plans was carried out following each session. Consideration was given to:

○ Group members' targets

○ The activities used (including the suitability of the levels worked at)

○ Progress made and issues raised

○ Environmental factors

○ Communication, interaction and behaviour of the group facilitators as well as interactions of group members

Working example 2 planning & running a group for members at the facilitating independence stage

This group was facilitated by a speech & language therapist and an occupational therapist. They both worked exclusively with young people with ASD and were experienced in running groups. Maria and Vishnu were well-known to the group facilitators from previous groups, but Brendan and Paul were less familiar to them. Here are their individual case studies.

BRENDAN is 15 years old and has been diagnosed with ASD. He lives with his mum, dad and younger sister and attends a mainstream school without additional educational support. This is his first experience of groupwork. His mum and dad are very anxious about him becoming more independent within the home and the wider community, for example, going to the shops, using public transport and preparing meals and hot drinks. Brendan, however, is keen to gain independent living skills within these areas, but has unrealistic expectations of his own abilities. For example, he feels that he would be able to create a complicated three-course meal because he has seen it being prepared once on television, even though he has had limited experience of using cookery equipment at school and at home.

MARIA is 16 years old, with a diagnosis of ASD. She lives with her mum and older brother, who also has a diagnosis of ASD. She attends a specialist education unit for young people with ASD where independent living skills are encouraged and developed. She has attended groupwork since the age of 11. Maria comes across as being very sociable and confident. She is able to plan activities but struggles to transfer this theory into practical 'real-life' situations and can become highly anxious — speaking loudly and fast and seeking a lot of physical reassurance from group facilitators — for example, linking arms. She lacks insight and awareness into how this behaviour is perceived by others.

VISHNU is 15 and has a diagnosis of ASD. He lives at home with his mum, dad, older brother and younger sister. He attends a mainstream school with no additional educational support. He has attended two previous blocks of groupwork, which Vishnu and his mum and dad felt were beneficial. He is very solitary and describes himself as having no friends at school. He has a number of special interests. His parents are aware of this and support him by taking him to clubs relating to his interests, for example, computer games and engineering.

PAUL is 15 and has recently been diagnosed with ASD. He lives with his mum and their two cats. He attends mainstream school with no additional educational support. He presents as a very articulate, capable and mature young person who recognises that he has difficulties and that he is attending the group to learn more about himself and his diagnosis of ASD. He wishes to identify coping strategies to help him to manage his difficulties and feelings in relation to his diagnosis.

Prior to the group starting, the group facilitators held an informal meeting with each set of parents, where they discussed the general aims of the group and completed the Parent/carer assessment profile (see Chapter 3). They then carried out the Self-assessment profile with each group member individually.

Following this, the group facilitators were able to discuss and evaluate each young person's suitability and readiness for the group and identify individual targets in consultation with the group member and their parent or carer. These targets were recorded on the Assessment summary sheet (see Chapter 3). Below are the targets for each group member.

Brendan's targets

Agreed targets (to be reviewed after every session)

1 To develop his experience of a range of community activities
2 To develop his awareness of his own limitations with regards to independent living skills
3 To develop his ability to recognise when he needs to ask for help with activities

Maria's targets

Agreed targets (to be reviewed after every session)

1 To develop her practical skills when carrying out community activities related to daily living
2 To promote her self-confidence during these activities
3 To develop specific coping strategies to manage her anxieties

Vishnu's targets

Agreed targets (to be reviewed after every session)

1 To promote his awareness of others' points of view
2 To develop his skills of negotiation, compromise and problem-solving
3 To develop his awareness and use of social conversation skills

Paul's targets

Agreed targets (to be reviewed after every session)

1 To promote his awareness of ASD relating to himself and others
2 To develop coping strategies in relation to the difficulties he identifies
3 To meet new friends

The group facilitators met before the start of the first group session to discuss possible activities and themes that would promote the group members' targets. The group facilitators agreed that the group members were all approaching or at the facilitating independence stage and, therefore, the group timetable should reflect their need to develop their independence skills and confidence in the community setting. The group facilitators went to the first session with their own ideas, but also used a Thought shower (Activity 33) to elicit the suggestions and opinions of the group. During the first session, the group facilitators and group members devised an eighteen-week group timetable which includes several planned community visits.

Each session lasted for one and a half hours, except for Session 15 as this needed extra time to allow for travel to the restaurant and possible delays in ordering/receiving the meal.

We have also provided an example session plan for Session 15 where the group had planned to go on the bus to a restaurant. The group facilitators met for an hour before the session to identify how to use the community visit to meet the group members' targets. It also gave them an opportunity to discuss any possible safety issues and ensure that a risk assessment had been completed.

Group timetable – eighteen weeks

LOCATION Hospital/community visit

DATE TIMETABLE COMPLETED 10.01.XX

GROUP FACILITATORS PRESENT Vanisha Kahn, occupational therapist
Penelope Court-Hampton, speech & language therapist

NAMES OF GROUPWORK PARTICIPANTS Brendan, Vishnu, Maria, Paul

Session number	Session focus
1	Getting to know one another; setting activities
2	ASD: thoughts, feelings and opinions
3	Plan bowling trip
4	Bowling trip
5	Debrief after bowling trip: how did it go?
6	Friendships/relationships
7	Identifying your sensory preferences: taste
8	Phone for a pizza
9	Videoing role play on bullying
10	Stereotypes
11	Plan for getting the bus to the beach
12	Go to beach on the bus
13	Debrief following bus trip to the beach: how did it go?
14	Plan for trip on the bus to a restaurant
15	Go to the restaurant on the bus
16	Debrief following bus trip to the restaurant: how did it go?
17	Produce leaflet about the group
18	Final debrief – how did all the sessions go? Bring in food for farewell party

Session plan sheet – facilitating independence stage

DATE OF SESSION 18.04.XX

LOCATION Meet at the SLT in the hospital. Get the bus from outside the hospital to the 'Old Italian' restaurant. Return on the bus to the hospital, where group members will be collected as usual.

SESSION START TIME 17.00   **SESSION END TIME** 19.30

GROUP FACILITATORS
Vanisha Kahn, occupational therapist
Penelope Court–Hampton, speech & language therapist

GENERAL AIMS OF THE SESSION
To access and use public transport (bus)
To go for a pizza at a local restaurant (session 15)

Activities	Estimated time
· Public transport (Community visit F) Encourage each group member to ask for their fare and pay as practised in Role plays (Activity 31) from last week's session.	n/a
· Going for a pizza (Community visit D) Help Vishnu to get involved in conversation. Promote choice-making with group members when ordering. Encourage them to think about sensory preferences (taste).	n/a

General note:
Watch out for Maria showing signs of anxiety by becoming loud and talking fast/seeking physical reassurance. Prompt Brendan if he looks like he is struggling to ask for help. Help Vishnu to get involved in conversations.

Session plan sheet –
facilitating independence stage

COMMENTS (to be completed after peer review)

RESOURCES NEEDED

Signed consent form, funding, bus timetable

After the session, the group facilitators met to discuss and record how it went. They discussed each group member in turn and recorded the main things they had observed about them during the session. These observations were recorded on the Session record sheet (Appendix XIII) and used to review the group members' targets and alter them if necessary. We have provided a summary of the key points from the session record sheets of each group member below.

They also carried out a peer review to analyse the behaviour, communication and interactive styles of the group facilitators to identify any factors that may have significantly influenced the group members' performance. This was recorded in the 'Comments' section on the group session plan and used to modify the group facilitators' approach as required. We have provided a summary of the key points raised during peer review for each group member where relevant to illustrate important issues.

Summary of Session record sheet for Brendan

Despite his initial confidence from practice during the Role plays (Activity 31) in the previous group session, Brendan required support to ask and pay for his bus ticket. He was quiet and withdrawn throughout the journey, despite a number of attempts by the other group members to engage him in conversation. Brendan was, however, able to identify the correct bus stop and encouraged the others to get off. At the restaurant, Brendan struggled to choose what he wanted to eat. With support, he was able to choose a pizza but insisted on ordering a pudding designed for two to share. On the journey back, he complained of feeling nauseous.

Brendan's behaviour during the visit led the group facilitators to alter his targets. They felt that some issues had emerged in the session that would benefit from more specific targeting in the following group sessions and community visits, in particular the need to develop coping strategies and make appropriate choices. These revised targets were added to the Assessment summary sheet and Session record sheet.

Revised targets for Brendan

Agreed targets (to be reviewed after every session)

1 To explore coping strategies when things do not go to plan
2 To continue to promote his self-confidence and experience of community activities
3 To develop his own awareness of appropriate choice-making at a restaurant

Summary of key points from peer review

Peer review relating to Brendan focused on discussion about how appropriate it was to try to find out if anything was troubling him in situ or whether to wait until a later session. It was agreed that Brendan did not appear to be in a mood to tolerate intervention at the time and it was best left to a later date.

Summary of Session record sheet for Maria

Maria coped well with asking and paying for her ticket on the bus. She articulated how much she had been looking forward to the trip for the pizza. During the journey, she talked very fast and loudly. At the restaurant, she had no difficulties in making a choice and offered to place the order for the group with the waiter. However, when the waiter arrived to take the order, Maria became highly anxious, fidgety and was unable to remember the order. She told the group facilitators that she could not place the order. Maria remained loud and unsettled, and was unaware of how her behaviour was affecting others in the restaurant.

Maria's behaviour in the session prompted the group facilitators to alter her targets. Her changes in speech rate and volume were felt to be priorities, and the group facilitators talked about possible activities that would help her to identify these and to develop coping strategies. The group facilitators also discussed the need to promote Maria's self-confidence at all times. These amended targets were recorded on the Assessment summary sheet and Session record sheet.

Revised targets for Maria

Agreed targets (to be reviewed after every session)

1 To develop her awareness of volume/rate of speech and her levels of activity
2 To explore appropriate coping strategies to manage these
3 To develop her self-confidence during practical activities

Summary of key points from peer review

Following peer review, it was suggested that when Maria became very anxious in future sessions, one group facilitator would take her away from the group and encourage her to think about some of the coping strategies that they would be helping her to develop.

Summary of Session record sheet for Vishnu

Vishnu mumbled when asking for his bus ticket and the driver had to ask him to speak up. Vishnu repeated his request in the same way, showing that he required support from the group facilitators. At the restaurant, the group decided to order a starter to share. Vishnu was happy with the choice of garlic bread but wanted to add cheese to this. The rest of the group did not want the cheese. Vishnu appeared to become quite angry and frustrated with the group members and facilitators, despite them trying to talk to Vishnu about why they did not want cheese. For the rest of the session, he became withdrawn and directed conversation to one of the group facilitators about his special interests and the choice of starter.

After evaluating his performance on the group trip it was felt that Vishnu's targets remained appropriate for the next session.

Summary of key points from peer review

Peer review focused on how to approach Vishnu when the group members' choice did not fit in with his own. It was suggested that one group facilitator should continue to try to talk about this with him on a one-to-one basis, and to discuss possible resolutions when disagreements arose.

Summary of Session record sheet for Paul

Paul is used to using public transport independently and had no difficulties on the bus to the restaurant. He ordered his pizza without support. When it was late coming from the kitchen, Paul used inappropriate ways of dealing with this situation, for example, clicking his fingers and being aggressive towards the waiters. The group facilitators asked him whether his actions were the best way to deal with the situation and discussed appropriate alternatives. Paul then put this into practice and got his pizza.

Following discussion of how the session went for Paul, the group facilitators decided to keep his targets the same.

Summary of key points from peer review

In peer review, the group facilitators agreed that the session had gone well for Paul. They felt that they had both handled the situation well in discussing appropriate ways for him to deal with the situation of the late pizzas, as he was able to put their advice into practice.

Below is the Session plan for Session 16, outlining planned activities. It also has details of things the group facilitators need to look out for following their observations and peer review of the trip to the restaurant.

Session plan sheet – facilitating independence stage

DATE OF SESSION 25.04.XX **LOCATION** SLT room in hospital

SESSION START TIME 17.00 **SESSION END TIME** 19.30

GROUP FACILITATORS Vanisha Kahn, occupational therapist
Penelope Court-Hampton, speech & language therapist

GENERAL AIMS OF THE SESSION To 'debrief' the group following last week's
community visit (session 16)

Activities	Estimated time
• Prepare a snack whilst completing Good and bad things from the week (Activity 28) at Level 2. This will give the group an opportunity to settle into the session and discuss any issues that have arisen over the past week with the group facilitators and peers. Encourage Maria to make the snack to help develop her confidence with practical activities.	
• Friendship darts (Activity 6) at Level 1, using the theme of positive/ negative things that happened during last week's pizza outing. The group facilitators will join in and contribute with their observations about how it went to prompt group members if they struggle to think of things or come out with unrealistic or unusual ideas.	
• Role plays (Activity 31) at Level 1. Group facilitators will choose one situation relating to each group member and the group role plays this, eg, choosing too much food (Brendan), talking too loudly (Maria), ordering food (Vishnu) and complaining (Paul). Be aware of any sensitivities that arose from the Friendship darts activity. If a group member will not accept that this was a problem for them, consider an alternative.	
• Discuss with the group options of activity choices and themes for the next session (refer back to 18-week plan). Encourage Vishnu to negotiate.	

Session plan sheet – facilitating independence stage

COMMENTS (to be completed after peer review)

RESOURCES NEEDED

Snacks, dart board and darts

The same process of reflection and modification of targets and the session plans was carried out following every session. Consideration was given to:

- Group members' targets
- The activities used (including the suitability of any levels worked at)
- Progress made and issues raised
- Environmental factors
- Communication, interaction and behaviour of the group facilitators as well as interactions of group members

Activities

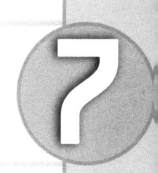

T he activities in this book can be used to develop a range of skills across seven key developmental areas. Each activity included has a list of possible targets that are grouped to show how they could meet the young person's needs in the seven key development areas described in Chapter 1. In addition, four sub-categories have been used to clarify which aspects of behavioural and emotional development some of the activities could be used for. The targets are grouped into the following. The four sub-categories appear at the end of the list.

- Language and communication skills
- Socialisation
- Leisure time
- Sensory issues
- Motor skills
- Behaviour
- Emotional development
- Understanding of diagnosis
- Transitions
- Self-awareness and the development of coping strategies
- Independent living skills

These targets are examples of the way in which we have used the activities within our groups, but are by no means the only skills that can be developed using the activity. Indeed, the main emphasis of our approach is to be flexible and alter activities according to the needs of the group at that time. You will be able to use the activities as we suggest or adapt them to suit the needs of your group members.

Activity levels

The activities are described at several levels of usage. These levels offer ideas of how an activity can be differentiated and graded according to the group members' level of functioning. They also enable the activities to be used repeatedly in different ways and with different expectations. Some group members may attend several groups between the ages of 11 and 16, and reuse of activities in a different way builds on the skills acquired in earlier groups.

How to use the activities

Some groups approaching a transition point (eg, transfer to secondary school at age 11) may benefit from a combination of activities from this book and the previous book in the series (5–11 years). A number of the activities appear in both books. This recognises the benefit of and need for repetition for these young people in helping them to establish skills. The activities are not exactly the same, however, but add new levels of sophistication as they progress through the age levels. For example, in this book, Interviews (Activity 3) plans to build on the skills of turn-taking, asking questions, forming friendships and recognising similarities and differences in others that were introduced in activities in the previous book, but aims to develop them at a higher level where group members are encouraged to evaluate their own performance through the use of video.

The activities are ordered into an activities index, which can be found on the following two pages. They are arranged into the general themes in which we would tend to use them (eg, warm-up/round-up activities, motor/physical activities), but can and should be used flexibly according to the needs of your group. For example, some of the group games such as Salt jars (Activity 8) and Pool (Activity 9) can be used for problem-solving and emotions/mental health in addition to the suggested theme of learning about ourselves. The key is to organise the work space and sequence the activities in a way that works for your group.

Within the activities index, we have also recommended an age range to assist you in selecting activities. The *emerging independence* stage is for 11–13 years and the *facilitating independence* stage is for 14–16 years. The age ranges are a guide and should be applied carefully and used with discretion, remembering that an activity suggested for the facilitating independence stage may also be appropriate for group members still in the emerging independence stage. Within the index, we have indicated the levels of the activities that would be expected at each stage.

Cautionary note

Some activities are highly emotive and address issues around group members' mental health. We have indicated this in the text with the symbol ⚠ at the top of the activities. We feel that it is important to highlight the need to read the Top tips for these activities thoroughly before commencing the activity. It may be more appropriate for professionals new to the field of ASD to refer these young people to a more experienced colleague.

○ Activities index

Activity number	Activity	Levels suitable for the emerging independence stage	Levels suitable for the facilitating independence stage	Page number
Warm-up/round-up games				
1	Parachute games	All	All	102
Learning about ourselves				
2	People bingo	All	All	104
3	Interviews	1–3	All	106
4	Show and tell	1–2	All	109
5	Feely bags	All	All	111
6	Friendship darts	All	All	113
7	Compliments	All	All	115
8	Salt jars	All	All	116
9	Pool	All	All	118
10	Tasting	All	All	120
11	Knowing your preferences	All	All	122
12	Hangman	All	All	124
13	Just a minute	1–3	All	126
Motor/physical activities				
14	Circuits	1–4	All	128
15	Obstacle course	1–4	All	131
16	Relays	1–3	All	134
Group games				
17	Kim's game	All	All	136
18	Spot the differences	All	All	138
19	Mimes	All	All	140
20	Charades	1	All	142
21	Say the picture	All	All	144
22	Who am I?	All	All	146
23	Zoo	All	All	148

Activity number	Activity	Levels suitable for the emerging independence stage	Levels suitable for the facilitating independence stage	Page number
Working as a team				
24	Making sandwiches	All	All	150
25	Treasure hunt	1–4	All	152
26	Token challenge	1	All	155
27	Group picnic game	1–2	All	157
Problem-solving				
28	Good and bad things from the week	1–2	All	160
29	Leaflets/questionnaires	All	All	162
30	Debates	1	All	164
31	Role plays	1–2	All	166
32	Quizzes	1–2	All	169
33	Thought showers	All	All	171
Emotions/mental health				
34	Act out emotions	All	All	173
35	Planets	1–2	All	175
36	Emotional thermometers	All	All	177
37	Life maps	All	All	180
38	Power circles	1	All	182
39	The colour of feelings	All	All	184
40	What's in my head?	1	All	186

Activity 1
Parachute games

 Equipment Parachute

 Targets

LANGUAGE/ COMMUNICATION	• To develop turn-taking
	• To develop attention and listening skills
	• To promote decision/choice-making
	• To develop auditory memory
SOCIALISATION	• To learn group members' names
	• To promote appropriate eye contact with other group members
SENSORY	• To calm or alert (depending on the individual's sensory profile)
MOTOR	• To develop shoulder stability
	• To develop spatial awareness
	• To develop motor planning
EMOTIONS	• To develop group cohesion and trust

 Top tips

○ Be aware of safety issues. Some group members will collide with each other. Think: is this a behaviour, motor planning or sensory issue?

○ Watch for sensory overload. You may need to control the speed of the parachute to prevent flapping.

○ You may need to do a round robin of names before beginning the activity as some group members may struggle to remember names.

○ If group members are struggling to remember names, encourage them to ask. You may need to prompt: 'What can you ask to find out their name?' If they cannot think of anything to say, ask them to copy you saying 'What is your name?'

○ Make sure everyone says hello to each individual.

○ Observe their ability to lift the parachute and give eye contact.

P Routledge
Taylor & Francis Group

○ When encouraging eye contact, explain why it is important to give it in this situation.

○ We often use this activity at the beginning and end of the group session, as it clearly defines the boundaries of the session to the group members. When using it to end the group, we say 'Goodbye___' instead of 'Hello___'.

○ When ending the session with this activity, it can be used to calm or alert the group members, depending on their presentation. For example, if the session has included lots of table-top activities, a loud goodbye can alert them for leaving. However, if the group have become very active as a result of the group session content and are difficult to focus, a quiet whispered goodbye, without doing Levels 2 and 3, can help to calm them.

Activity levels

Level 1

○ The group members stand in a circle.

○ Each group member holds onto the parachute edge with two hands.

○ The facilitator explains that, after the count of three, everyone will lift up the parachute and one group member will say 'Hello___' to a chosen individual (eg, 'Hello David'). Stress that it is important to try to look at this individual. They will then put the parachute back down again.

○ Repeat until everyone has had a turn.

Level 2

○ Stand in a circle.

○ Each group member holds onto the edge of the parachute with both hands.

○ Explain that, after the count of three, the parachute will be raised. The group facilitator will call out two names and those people will swap places.

○ Allow time for the individuals to swap places, then bring the parachute back down again.

○ Repeat until everyone has had a few goes.

Level 3

○ Let the individual group members choose someone to swap with them.

○ Ensure that everyone has a turn.

Groupwork for Children with ASD Ages 11–16 © A Eggett, K Old, LA Davidson & C Howe 2008

Activity 2
People bingo

Equipment   A prepared people bingo sheet for each group member (see Appendices XIV and XV)

Pens/pencils

Targets

LANGUAGE/ COMMUNICATION	• To develop the ability to ask and answer questions • To promote recording – pictorial or written • To promote turn-taking
SOCIALISATION	• To develop awareness of others' appearance, personal characteristics and interests • To practise appropriate initiation of conversation
LEISURE TIME AND INTERESTS	• To explore others' interests and hobbies
EMOTIONS	• To develop group cohesion and trust • To explore a range of emotions

Top tips

○ You may need to explain the meaning of 'appearance'. This is the easiest concept to begin with as these characteristics are visual. Move on to other characteristics (eg, interests) at a later time.

○ Encourage questions. At first, you may need to model or say the question and get the individual to repeat what you have said.

○ Model and allow alternative ways of recording (eg, drawing).

○ Be prepared to give some members one-to-one attention during this activity.

Activity levels

Level 1

○ Give each group member a bingo sheet.

○ Explain that they are going to play bingo with people's appearance instead of numbers.

This page may be photocopied for instructional use only. Groupwork for Children with ASD Ages 11–16 © A Eggett, K Old, LA Davidson & C Howe 2008

○ Explain to the group members that they need to look at the themes on their sheets and find someone in the group with those characteristics.

○ Encourage them to look at people appropriately. They may have to get up and wander around the room and ask questions.

○ Once they have found someone with a particular characteristic, they record that person's name on the sheet.

○ They continue until the sheet is completed.

Level 2

○ Introduce more complex ideas (such as interests, emotions, experiences, hobbies).

Routledge
Taylor & Francis Group
ROUTLEDGE

Activity 3
Interviews

Equipment   Prepared interview sheets (see Appendix XVI)
Blank interview sheets (see Appendix XVII)
Video camera
Television with video player

Targets

LANGUAGE/ COMMUNICATION	• To ask and answer questions • To promote recording skills • To promote turn-taking
SOCIALISATION	• To promote friendship-making skills • To develop awareness of others' appearance, personal characteristics and interests • To increase awareness of similarities and differences with peers
LEISURE TIME AND INTERESTS	• To explore others' hobbies and interests
UNDERSTANDING OF DIAGNOSIS	• To promote awareness of their diagnosis

Top tips

For all levels

○ Position pairs according to sensory preferences (eg, in quieter parts of the room, at a desk not on the floor).

○ A high level of one-to-one support may be needed for less able pairs.

○ Modelling is essential for this activity. Model how to give feedback and be prepared to give lots of prompts.

○ Allow for different methods of recording (eg, drawing).

Routledge
Taylor & Francis Group

For levels 4 and 5

○ Gain consent from parents and carers and the group members for videoing.

○ A room with a camera, recording facilities, television and video are needed at these levels.

○ Some group members may need a high level of adult supervision to operate equipment. Be aware of any health and safety issues relating to the equipment being used.

○ Some group members may find being filmed anxiety provoking. This needs to be handled sensitively. A 'behind camera' role may be more suitable for these individuals until they are more relaxed and confident.

○ At Level 4, some group members may need a specific target to look for when analysing themselves (eg, eye contact, turn-taking or body language). You may need to explain what these things are and why they are important for successful communication.

○ The interviews can be used to explore individuals' awareness of their diagnosis. The group facilitators should have prepared interview questions. Examples of questions you may wish to include are: 'Have you heard of ASD before?', 'What do you think your difficulties are?', 'Do you know anyone else with ASD?', 'How does it impact on your home/school life?', 'How long have you had ASD?'

 Activity levels

Level 1

○ Discuss with the group any interviews that they may have seen on television. Explain they are going to interview each other.

○ Talk about meeting people for the first time and what things they may want to find out about them.

○ Facilitators role play an interview.

○ Put group members into ability-matched pairs.

○ Give each pair a prepared interview sheet.

○ Get them to take turns to be the interviewer asking the questions and the interviewee answering.

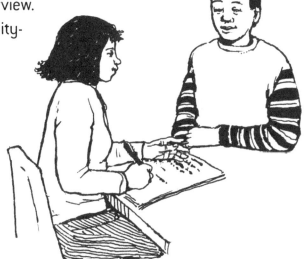

Routledge Taylor & Francis Group

○ Get the interviewer to record their partner's answers.

○ Group members then feed back what they have found out to the rest of the group.

Level 2

○ Decrease prompts.

○ Add more questions and get the group members to think of two of their own.

Level 3

○ Get the group members to design their own interview sheets.

Level 4

○ Record the interviews using a video camera.

○ Get the group members to watch back their interview in their pairs.

○ Discuss and reflect on their performance, encouraging feedback (eg, non-verbal communication, volume).

Level 5

○ Group members not involved in the interview may take on the role of operating the equipment, with each group member taking a turn. You may need to model this first. It is important that the interviewer and interviewee are comfortable with other people observing and commenting on their performance.

Routledge
Taylor & Francis Group

Activity 4
Show and tell

Equipment   Show and tell letter to take home (see Appendix XVIII)

Targets

LANGUAGE/ COMMUNICATION	• To promote turn-taking skills • To develop expressive language skills • To promote asking of appropriate questions
SOCIALISATION	• To link home with another setting
LEISURE TIME AND INTERESTS	• To explore others' hobbies and interests
EMOTIONS	• To establish relationships • To promote a sense of trust and belonging

Top tips

○ Gain consent from parents and carers for the videoing of this activity.

○ It is important to give the letter to parents and carers at the emerging independence stage, as the group members may not be relied on to remember by themselves. This level of support should be reduced as group members move towards the facilitating independence stage.

○ Give guidelines about the practicalities of bringing objects to group members (eg, a photograph of their dog is more appropriate than bringing the dog to the group).

○ Some group members may need encouragement to listen to others when they are presenting their item.

○ Dissuade negative comments.

○ Encourage relevant questions. Discuss why questions are/are not relevant.

○ Be prepared to point out when a group member has gone on for too long. This can lead to discussion about how you can tell when a person is not interested in what you have to say (eg, by observing their body language).

Groupwork for Children with ASD Ages 11–16 © A Eggett, K Old, LA Davidson & C Howe 2008

Routledge
Taylor & Francis Group
ROUTLEDGE

○ Allow plenty of time for this activity at Levels 2 and 3.

○ Some group members may find being filmed anxiety provoking. This will need to be handled sensitively and group members should be positively encouraged to participate. If this is too difficult, a 'behind camera' role may be more suitable for these individuals until they are more relaxed and confident.

Activity levels

Level 1

○ Hand out the letter to parents and carers at the session before you intend to do this activity. When you hand the letters out, explain to group members that you want them to bring something special in next week to talk to the group about.

○ Each group member takes it in turn to talk to the rest of the group about the object they have brought in and why it is special to them.

○ Other group members are encouraged to ask questions.

Level 2

○ Get group members to produce a two-minute presentation on their chosen subject. This can be done with support within the group or given as a homework task for them to present next session.

○ Encourage questions from group members following the presentations.

Level 3

○ The group facilitator videos each group member's presentation.

○ The group watch the videos together and discuss each presentation. Encourage positive and appropriate feedback (eg, staying on topic, answering questions appropriately).

Activity 5
Feely bags

Equipment
Several bags or boxes
Different tactile materials (eg, rice, sand, shaving foam, foam shapes, lentils, pasta, wood shavings, polystyrene balls, feathers, cotton wool)
A list of bag/box contents for each group member
Small items (eg, a rubber, toy car, Lego, crayon, coin, comb, toothbrush)

Targets

LANGUAGE/ COMMUNICATION	• To develop expressive language skills
SENSORY	• To develop sensory skills
MOTOR	• To develop fine motor skills

Top tips

○ Check the safety of all equipment.

○ Be aware of sensory issues. Some young people may have an over-responsive sensory system, which can lead to gagging or even vomiting.

○ If a young person is very reluctant to participate due to sensory issues or low self-esteem, do not force them to have a go. This activity requires a high level of sensitivity and support when encouraging group members to participate.

○ If a group member cannot name the thing in the bag/box, get them to draw a picture or describe it (eg, slimy, rough, dry).

○ This activity lends itself to themes (such as going to a new school or Halloween) by hiding objects relevant to that theme.

Activity levels

Level 1

○ Set up the bags/boxes, each with a different tactile material inside. Mark each bag/box with a number.

This page may be photocopied for instructional use only. *Groupwork for Children with ASD Ages 11–16* © A Eggett, K Old, LA Davidson & C Howe 2008

○ Have a list of the materials in the bags/boxes for each group member.

○ Each group member has a turn at putting their hand in each bag/box.

○ They then record on their list the bag/box number next to the material they think is inside.

○ After everyone has had a turn, compare answers and show the contents of the bags/boxes.

Level 2

○ Get group members to write down what they think is in each bag/box without having a list.

Activity 6
Friendship darts

 Equipment   Magnetic/sticky dartboard

 Targets

LANGUAGE/ COMMUNICATION	• To promote listening skills • To promote turn-taking
SOCIALISATION	• To develop awareness of the qualities of friendship • To build group trust
MOTOR	• To develop hand–eye co-ordination
EMOTIONS	• To develop awareness of emotions • To develop awareness of others' emotions
SELF- AWARENESS AND COPING STRATEGIES	• To promote identification of appropriate coping strategies

 Top tips

- Ensure that all group members stand well out of the range of the dartboard to avoid the risk of accidents.
- Each group member's motor skills will influence how far away they can be from the board to succeed in hitting it.
- Dissuade negative comments about people's throwing ability.
- This activity can be used for other subjects apart from friendship (eg, likes/ dislikes, hobbies, school, anger management).

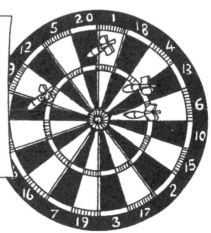

Black =
Good things
about school
White =
Things I
don't like
about school

Groupwork for Children with ASD Ages 11–16 © A Eggett, K Old, LA Davidson & C Howe 2008

Routledge
Taylor & Francis Group
ROUTLEDGE

○ Encourage group discussion around the chosen theme and relate this to personal situation-based experiences (eg, an incident at school). Discuss the suitability of the group members' coping strategies in these situations.

Activity levels

Level 1

○ Set up the dartboard.

○ Explain that, if the group members hit one colour, they need to think of a positive quality associated with friendship; the other colour a negative trait not associated with good friendships (eg, tells tales).

○ Each group member takes it in turn to throw a dart and think of an idea.

○ Encourage discussion about their own experiences and problem-solving of any issues raised.

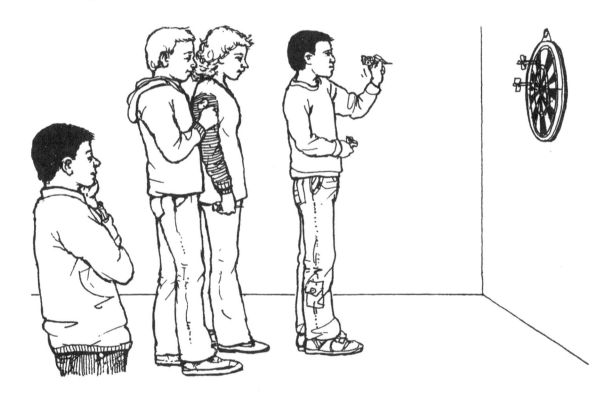

Activity 7
Compliments

Equipment   None

Targets

LANGUAGE/ COMMUNICATION	• To promote choice/decision-making • To promote conversational skills (eg, relevancy) • To develop expressive communication skills • To develop turn-taking
EMOTIONS	• To promote trust among group members

Top tips

○ Be aware of negative comments. Always explain why they are not appropriate, stressing how it makes the person receiving the 'compliment' feel.

○ Some group members may find it difficult to express themselves in this activity. To boost self-esteem, ensure that you praise positive comments.

○ Some group members may always pick the same person, or may struggle to pick one person to give a compliment to. To avoid this, you could write group members' names down on slips of paper and get them to pick names out of a hat.

○ It can be useful to write down these compliments to review with group members at a later date.

Activity levels

Level 1

○ Explain to the group that they are going to practise giving and receiving compliments. You may need to explain the meaning of a 'compliment'.

○ Model a positive and negative comment about the appearance/personality of the group facilitator to give examples of appropriate comments.

○ Group members take it in turns to pick another group member and practise giving compliments to them.

This page may be photocopied for instructional use only. *Groupwork for Children with ASD Ages 11–16* © A Eggett, K Old, LA Davidson & C Howe 2008

Activity 8
Salt jars

Equipment   Small glass or plastic jars or bottle with lids
Salt
Pastels
Paper
Aprons

Targets

EMOTIONS	
	• To promote a sense of trust and rapport within the group
	• To encourage self-disclosure
	• To encourage expression of feelings, emotions and opinions

Top tips

○ This activity can be based on a range of interests/hobbies including friendship qualities and emotions.

○ Depending on the theme, the facilitators will need to create a safe environment in order to encourage self-expression. Be aware of more sensitive topics.

○ This is quite a nice 'getting to know you' or round-up activity for the group.

Activity levels

Level 1

○ Explain to the group that they are going to make a salt jar. Have one almost completed and model its making.

○ Select a theme to work on (eg, friendship).

○ Ask the group to identify different qualities that a person may have related to this theme (eg, kindness, sharing, trustworthy, good listener). Write these down on a piece of paper.

○ The group members then chose a pastel colour that they feel represents each quality (eg, kind = yellow, fun = red).

Routledge
Taylor & Francis Group

- Provide each group member with five separate sheets of paper. Get them to write one quality per piece of paper in the identified colour (ie, 'kind' in yellow pastel, 'fun' in red pastel).
- Give each group member a jar filled with salt.
- Get them to divide the salt from the jar between the five pieces of paper. This means that each piece of paper will have a small pile of salt in the middle of it. Different qualities may be allocated different amounts of salt depending on the group members' feelings.
- When salt is rubbed over with a pastel, it will turn the colour of that pastel. The group members take the corresponding colour for the identified quality on their piece of paper and colour the salt piled in the centre of the paper with that pastel.
- Once all the piles of salt have been coloured in by the pastel, the individuals pour the salt into the jars in layers (eg, 'kind' first, 'fun' next).
- Encourage discussion about the balance of colours in their jars.
- Group members can take their jar home if they wish.

This has been adapted from an original activity. Written by Diana Crossley, designed and illustrated by Kate Sheppard. *Muddles, Puddles and Sunshine*, 2000. © Published by Hawthorn Press. Adapted with permission. www.hawthornpress.com

Groupwork for Children with ASD Ages 11–16 © A Eggett, K Old, LA Davidson & C Howe 2008

Routledge
Taylor & Francis Group
ROUTLEDGE

Activity 9
Pool

 Equipment   Pool table, cues and balls. (Depending on space and facilities, some venues may have access to a full-size pool/snooker table. If yours does not, you could source a portable table-top sized pool table from a local toy shop.)
Paper and pens

 Targets

LANGUAGE/ COMMUNICATION	• To promote listening skills • To promote turn-taking • To promote the ability to follow verbal instructions
SOCIALISATION	• To identify qualities of friendships • To promote teamwork skills • To promote the ability to follow rules • To identify likes/dislikes • To raise awareness of their fellow peers' likes/dislikes
MOTOR	• To promote hand–eye co-ordination • To promote fine motor skills • To promote the development of motor planning
EMOTIONS	• To promote identification of a range of emotions • To develop the ability to identify their own emotions • To develop the ability to link emotions with real-life situations
INDEPENDENT LIVING SKILLS	• To explore themes related to independent living skills
SELF- AWARENESS AND COPING STRATEGIES	• To begin to identify and explore appropriate coping strategies • To recognise and identify inappropriate coping strategies • To promote the use of appropriate coping strategies in real-life situations
UNDERSTANDING OF DIAGNOSIS	• To increase awareness, knowledge and understanding of ASD
TRANSITIONS	• To explore and discuss issues about transitions

Routledge
Taylor & Francis Group

Top tips

- Be aware of the safety issues when using pool cues.
- Some group members may find it physically difficult to hold the cue and co-ordinate potting the balls. Ensure that a supportive environment is maintained for these individuals.
- This activity can be used to explore a range of themes, for example, anger, emotions, community visits, teamwork (divide the group into teams for this), losing, diagnosis, transitions and coping strategies.

Activity levels

Level 1

- Set up the pool table.
- Explain to group members that they are going to play pool with a difference.
- Explain the rules: that if they pot a yellow ball, the group members have to share something they like associated with the chosen theme. If they pot a red ball, they share something they do not like.

Routledge
Taylor & Francis Group
ROUTLEDGE

Activity 10
Tasting

Equipment   A variety of foods to taste (such as fruit, crisps, sweets)
Pens/paper
Blindfolds (optional)
Plates/bowls

Targets

LANGUAGE/ COMMUNICATION	• To develop attention and listening skills • To develop vocabulary related to tasting • To record information appropriately • To promote turn-taking
SOCIALISATION	• To create a sense of fun and ease within the group
SENSORY	• To explore tactile, oral and gustatory senses • To identify likes and dislikes
EMOTIONS	• To be aware of emotional reactions to different tastes
SELF- AWARENESS AND COPING STRATEGIES	• To increase a sense of awareness of taste, smell and texture • To explore and develop coping strategies in relation to likes and dislikes

Top tips

- Check consent forms for any allergies.
- Beware of sensory issues relating to tasting. Some individuals may have an over-responsive sensory system which can lead to gagging or vomiting.
- Be aware of sensory issues and anxiety issues relating to wearing a blindfold/ closing their eyes.
- If a group member does not want to participate in the activity, do not force this, but do encourage them to have a try.
- Discourage shouting out. Try to stress that it is a secret activity until the end when the tastes are revealed by the facilitators.
- Encourage group members to be positive towards one another.
- Some group members may need help to grade tastes.

At Level 1, crisps are useful as you cannot distinguish between tastes by sight.

Activity levels

Level 1

Before group members arrive, set up four bowls with four different tastes (eg, four different flavours of crisps).

Each group member has a pen and paper and writes the numbers one to four down the left-hand side.

One of the bowls is placed in the middle and each group member has a taste.

They then write down what they think the flavour is (eg, salt and vinegar, cheese and onion).

Level 2

Blindfold group members before they do the tasting.

Level 3

Group members rate the tastes in order of preference.

Level 4

The group members create a group profile of likes and dislikes, for example, by making a graph, histogram or pie chart representing the number of group members that like/dislike a certain taste.

Level 5

Another useful activity is to write an individual profile of taste preferences. This helps group members to increase their own awareness of their likes and dislikes and to make appropriate choices. This can also be used to discuss coping strategies to help them to manage social situations (eg, going to a restaurant).

Activity 11
Knowing your preferences

 Equipment Selection of sensory equipment (see Appendix XX)
A notebook and pen for each group member

 Targets

LANGUAGE/ COMMUNICATION	• To develop reporting skills
	• To develop recording information in different ways
SOCIALISATION	• To develop negotiation skills
SENSORY	• To explore the sensory systems within our bodies
	• To explore our individual preferences within these sensory systems
EMOTIONS	• To explore how sensory input impacts on emotions
SELF-AWARENESS AND COPING STRATEGIES	• To increase self-awareness of their own sensory behaviours and thresholds
	• To explore coping strategies to manage sensory issues
INDEPENDENT LIVING	• To understand the impact on daily living of sensory issues

 Top tips

○ Be aware of any aversions to sensory stimuli (eg, noise) and allow the group members to opt out of exploration if they need to. If they feel uncomfortable, they can simply discuss their preferences with their peers.

○ Adverse reactions to sensory input can occur for a few hours after exposure. Parents and carers need to be advised about this so that they can manage these and bring any concerns to the group facilitators' attention.

○ Allow for breaks if the group members become overly stimulated or uncomfortable.

○ This activity could be carried out each session, focusing on one sense at a time, until all seven have been explored.

Routledge
Taylor & Francis Group
ROUTLEDGE

A book can be created for each individual group member, listing each sensory system, the types of stimuli they may encounter, their likes and dislikes and coping strategies to deal with them.

Activity levels

Level 1

- The group members are asked to think about the different senses (taste, smell, sight, hearing and touch).
- The additional senses of vestibular and proprioception (see Chapter 1) are included in the list and explained to the group members.
- Select one sense to explore in the session (eg, touch).
- A range of sensory stimuli relating to this sense are presented to the group (eg, brushes, slime, cooked cold pasta, jelly, cotton wool, fabrics).
- In their notebook, the group members record whether they like or dislike these particular sensory stimuli.
- The members are then asked to compare their own preferences with those of other members of the group.

Level 2

- As above, but encourage group members to grade the stimuli from favourite to least liked.
- Group members are encouraged to think of ways they can deal with uncomfortable stimuli and discuss appropriate coping strategies to manage these.
- The group member may record in their notebook each sensory system alongside any coping strategies that they have developed.

Routledge
Taylor & Francis Group

Activity 12
Hangman

Equipment   Prepared game cards labelled with words associated with the chosen theme (see the Activities card template Appendix XIX for photocopiable blank cards to write on)
Pens/pencils

Targets

LANGUAGE/ COMMUNICATION	• To develop the ability to interpret information and make predictions based on it • To promote recording – pictorial and/or written • To promote turn-taking
SOCIALISATION	• To develop awareness of others' appearance, personal characteristics and interests • To promote teamwork skills
LEISURE TIME AND INTERESTS	• To explore a range of interests and hobbies
EMOTIONS	• To develop group cohesion and trust • To explore a range of emotions
UNDERSTANDING OF DIAGNOSIS	• To promote awareness of their diagnosis of ASD

Top tips

- Some group members may need help with reading the words, preparing the word grid and creating the hangman illustration.
- Encourage sensitivity towards group members who find organising and recording information difficult.

Routledge
Taylor & Francis Group
ROUTLEDGE

Activity levels

Level 1

- Use a theme associated with issues that have been raised by individual group members (eg, making friends), group members' targets (eg, recognising emotions) or a forthcoming community visit (eg, to the cinema).
- Prepare a range of cards in advance labelled with different words written on that are related to the chosen theme.
- Each group member takes a turn to choose a game card. They need to work out how many letters are in the word and prepare the word grid to fill in as the others try to guess the word.
- The other members of the group take turns to guess the letters in the word and, ultimately, the word itself.
- The group member with the game card needs to fill in the word grid as letters are appropriately guessed and add to the hangman illustration when guesses are incorrect.

Level 2

- Encourage the group members to divide into two teams. Help them to negotiate how the group will be divided, which team will go first and the rules of the game (eg, the first team to get three wins).
- Each team takes a turn. The team nominates a member to choose the word and complete the word grid and hangman.
- Continue playing until one of the teams wins.

Level 3

- Encourage the group members to chose their own themes, identify associated words and, in teams, to prepare the game cards.

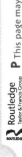
This page may be photocopied for instructional use only. *Groupwork for Children with ASD Ages 11–16* © A Eggett, K Old, LA Davidson & C Howe 2008

Routledge
Taylor & Francis Group

Activity 13
Just a minute

Equipment   Stop watch
Video camera
Television and video/DVD player

Targets

LANGUAGE/ COMMUNICATION	• To develop attention and listening skills
	• To develop the ability to ask and answer questions
	• To develop expressive language skills
SOCIALISATION	• To increase awareness of similarities and differences with peers
	• To develop awareness of others' appearance, personal characteristics and interests
LEISURE TIME AND INTERESTS	• To explore a range of interests and hobbies
EMOTIONS	• To develop group cohesion and trust
SELF- AWARENESS AND COPING STRATEGIES	• To explore and promote appropriate coping strategies (eg, time management)

Top tips

- Gain consent from parents and carers and the individuals for videoing at Levels 4 and 5.
- Initially, some members may require a long period for preparation – it may help to give them a topic to plan a talk about for presentation at the following group session.
- Model how to give feedback and ask appropriate questions.
- Some group members may find being filmed anxiety provoking. This needs to be handled sensitively. A 'behind camera' role may be more suitable for these individuals until they are more relaxed and confident.

Routledge
Taylor & Francis Group

At Level 4, some group members may need a specific target to look for when analysing themselves (eg, eye contact, turn-taking, body language). You may need to explain what these things are and why they are important for successful communication.

Some group members may need a high level of adult supervision to operate equipment. Be aware of any health and safety issues relating to the equipment being used.

Activity levels

Level 1

Each group member chooses a topic to talk to the rest of the group about. Often, this will be related to a special interest.

Allow the group members time to plan what they are going to talk about.

Each group member takes a turn at talking for one minute about their chosen topic to the rest of the group.

Level 2

Encourage more specific planning of the content of their talk (eg, making notes).

Group members are encouraged to talk for one minute without deviation from the subject or repetition of the content.

Other members of the group are encouraged to ask questions after the talk.

Level 3

Work towards group members being given a topic to talk about to extend their knowledge and interests. For example, if a group member is interested in computer games, encourage him to widen his topic by talking about something similar, like how computers benefit schools.

Some group members could be encouraged to plan and present a talk in pairs.

Level 4

Film the talks.

Get group members to watch their own presentation.

Encourage them to reflect on their performance (eg, on repetition or volume).

Level 5

Group members not involved in the presentation take on the role of operating the equipment, with each group member taking a turn with this. The presenting group member needs to feel comfortable with others observing and commenting on his presentation style at this level.

Groupwork for Children with ASD Ages 11–16 © A Eggett, K Old, LA Davidson & C Howe 2008

This page may be photocopied for instructional use only.

Routledge Taylor & Francis Group

Activity 14
Circuits

 Equipment See Appendix XXIV for a list of possible activities and equipment

 Targets

LANGUAGE/ COMMUNICATION	• To develop attention and listening skills
	• To follow visual and verbal instructions
SENSORY	• To develop sensory awareness
	• To develop orientation within the environment
MOTOR	• To develop gross motor skills
	• To develop motor planning skills
SOCIALISATION	• To encourage working as a team
	• To promote problem-solving
	• To consider others' views
	• To promote skills in compromise and negotiation
SELF-AWARENESS AND COPING STRATEGIES	• To promote the ability to reflect on one's own performance
	• To promote the development of coping strategies (eg, losing)

Top tips

○ Check the safety of all equipment.

○ Be aware of unsafe and unrealistic equipment choices by group members. Discuss and intervene as necessary.

○ Get the group to take their shoes or any loose clothing off. You may need to help some group members to take them off/put them back on.

○ Choose activities carefully. Provide supervision for more difficult equipment (eg, trampoline, wobble board).

○ Be aware of auditory defensiveness/unresponsiveness when using verbal instructions. Some group members may be better with a visual cue to move onto the next activity.

Be aware of any group members with low self-confidence. This is an activity that can be included in every session to build up confidence.

If you have group members with a poor attention span, circuits can be more successful than an obstacle course. Circuits involve the whole group working around the equipment in sequence, but at different time intervals, whereas an obstacle course involves group members completing the course with their peers waiting for a turn. Group members with a poor attention span may not cope with waiting, so circuits would be a better choice of activity.

A large mat or spots on the floor for group members to sit on will help them to focus when instructions are being given.

You may need to modify the time that some individuals spend on some equipment. Consider stamina, attention, impulsivity, general motor skills and confidence.

Select pairs/small groups carefully. Be aware of the skill mix and any personality clashes.

Model negotiation, compromise and teamwork.

At Level 5, this is a useful activity to video to reflect on teamwork skills.

Activity levels

Level 1

The group members sit together to listen to the instructions and watch a demonstration of the circuit.

Group facilitators set up the circuit in a circle, using the available equipment. There needs to be the same number of activities as there are group members.

Group facilitators demonstrate each activity.

Each group member is assigned to an activity by the group facilitator.

Each group member tries that activity for approximately two minutes.

The facilitators then cue the group members to move on to the next activity, using a clear and obvious auditory, visual and/or physical prompt (eg, shouting 'stop', raising a hand in a stop gesture and/or putting a hand on the group member's shoulder).

Continue until all the group members have tried each activity.

Level 2

Gradually fade out visual and physical prompts until you are using a more subtle auditory prompt to move group members along to the next activity (eg, whistle, music, rain stick).

This page may be photocopied for instructional use only. *Groupwork for Children with ASD Ages 11–16* © A Eggett, K Old, LA Davidson & C Howe 2008

Routledge
Taylor & Francis Group
ROUTLEDGE

Level 3

○ The group members choose one piece of equipment each from a selection to help to create the circuit prior to completing it. Encourage group members to consider their own and others' strengths and needs when choosing.

Level 4

○ Group members work in pairs/small groups to design their own circuit for the other pairs/small groups to carry out. Encourage pairs/small groups to consider others' strengths and needs when designing the circuit.

Level 5

○ Group members design the circuit as a whole group. Encourage negotiation and compromise amongst group members.

○ This can be videoed and watched back at the end to analyse teamworking skills.

Routledge
Taylor & Francis Group
ROUTLEDGE

Activity 15
Obstacle course

 Equipment   See Appendix XXIV for a list of possible activities and
equipment

Targets

LANGUAGE/ COMMUNICATION	• To follow verbal instructions
	• To develop attention and listening skills
	• To encourage turn-taking
SOCIALISATION	• To promote teamwork skills
	• To promote problem-solving
	• To promote skills in negotiation and compromise
	• To consider the views of others
SENSORY	• To promote the development of sensory skills
MOTOR	• To promote the development of motor planning
	• To promote the development of gross motor skills
SELF- AWARENESS AND COPING STRATEGIES	• To promote the ability to reflect on one's own performance
	• To promote the development of coping strategies (eg, losing)

Top tips

For all levels

Get the group to take off their shoes and any loose clothing. You may need to help some group members to take them off/put them back on.

This is a good activity to do before snack time as it helps to stimulate the group members and promotes organisational skills.

Use more or less equipment and grade the difficulty of the course depending on the ability of the group members.

Grade the amount of verbal and/or visual prompts to individual group members' needs.

Provide constant praise and positive encouragement to group members throughout the activity.

This page may be photocopied for instructional use only. Groupwork for Children with ASD Ages 11–16 © A Eggett, K Old, LA Davidson & C Howe 2008

Routledge
Taylor & Francis Group
ROUTLEDGE

- Encourage group members to cheer on their team mates. You may need to model this and get them to copy you.
- If carrying out this task on a weekly basis, the course may need to remain the same depending on ability levels. This presents an opportunity to bring in some variation by adding a surprise element and raising the challenge by adding another piece of equipment when appropriate.
- An element of teamwork can be added by timing the group's performance and recording this. This will help to increase awareness that things may go wrong, for example, one week the time may be slower than another.
- At Level 1, the emphasis is on negotiating the pieces of equipment, thus developing confidence and achievement. At Level 2, more complex motor and cognitive strategies are required. At Level 3, the element of planning, generating ideas and organisation skills are moving to the forefront.

Level 4

- A time limit of up to five minutes is given to design obstacle courses, as group members often lose track of time and can struggle to negotiate and compromise with their peers. Some group members may need help with generating ideas.
- Encourage and model positive negotiation and compromise skills. A high level of support may be needed for this until group members become more competent. At first, you may wish to group the young people to ensure an appropriate skill mix and group dynamic is achieved. This may be done subtly (eg, numbers under their chairs prior to the group starting).
- Be aware of dangerous or impossible obstacle courses created by group members, such as jumping off the trampoline onto the wobble board, standing on scooter boards or building unsafe structures to climb on. Discourage this and discuss why they are unsuitable.

For Level 5

- It may be useful to have a specific target that each group member needs to work on (eg, incorporating and listening to others' views, or agreeing who takes on different roles within the group).
- After watching the video, group members discuss ideas and strategies relating to good teamwork.
- A time limit may again need to be imposed on the obstacle course design.

Routledge
Taylor & Francis Group

Activity levels

Level 1

- Get the group members to sit together to listen to the instructions and watch a demonstration of the obstacle course.
- Set up the obstacle course with four selected activities.
- Explain and model the activities.
- The group members take it in turn to complete the obstacle course.

Level 2

- Increase the number of activities used.
- Ask one of the young people to demonstrate the activities.
- Use progressively difficult and contrasting equipment.

Level 3

- Ask each group member to choose a piece of equipment for making the course.
- Ask each group member to explain and model their piece of equipment to the rest of the group.

Level 4

- Divide the group into two teams or into pairs.
- Get them to design an obstacle course for the other team/pairs.
- The other team/pairs try out their course.

Level 5

- Video the Level 4 activity.
- Watch back the video and discuss group members' teamwork skills.

Routledge
Taylor & Francis Group

Activity 16
Relays

Groupwork for Children with ASD Ages 11–16 © A Eggett, K Old, LA Davidson & C Howe 2008

Equipment   See Appendix XXIV for a list of possible activities and equipment

Targets

LANGUAGE/ COMMUNICATION	• To promote turn-taking • To promote attention and listening skills • To follow verbal instructions
SOCIALISATION	• To promote and encourage teamworking • To promote problem-solving • To develop negotiation and compromise • To considers others' views
SENSORY	• To develop sensory awareness
MOTOR	• To develop motor planning
SELF-AWARENESS AND COPING STRATEGIES	• To promote the ability to reflect on one's own performance • To promote the development of coping strategies

Top tips

For all levels

- Get the group members to take off their shoes and any loose clothing. You may need to help some group members to take them off/put them back on.
- Be aware of sensory issues. This activity can get quite loud.
- Group facilitators select teams to encourage a skill mix.
- Provide visual markers (eg, mats, spots or hoops) to signal the start and end of the relay.
- Use visual markers to encourage team members to hold their position in line (eg, spots).
- Relays can be themed (eg, dressing up or collecting objects to make a picture associated with a chosen topic).

Routledge
Taylor & Francis Group

Encourage team members to support their team mates. You may need to explain why this is beneficial and model this.

For Level 4

It may be useful to have a specific target that each group member needs to work on (eg, incorporating and listening to others' views or agreeing who takes on different roles within the group).

After watching the video, group members could discuss ideas and strategies relating to good teamwork.

Activity levels

Level 1

Divide the group into two teams.

Set up and model the relay. Explain that team members take turns to complete the course. The first team to have all its members finish the course is the winner.

Carry out the relay.

Level 2

With support, allow group members to form their own team order.

Level 3

With maximum support, the teams design their own relays.

Level 4

Group facilitators video relays from Levels 2 and 3.

The group watch back the videos and discuss their performance.

Routledge
Taylor & Francis Group

P This page may be photocopied for instructional use only. *Groupwork for Children with ASD Ages 11–16* © A Eggett, K Old, LA Davidson & C Howe 2008

Activity 17
Kim's game

Equipment   A flat surface (eg, a tray or table)
A variety of objects
A cloth large enough to completely cover the objects

Targets

LANGUAGE/ COMMUNICATION	• To recall and describe a list of objects
	• To develop vocabulary
	• To develop attention and listening skills
	• To develop turn-taking
SENSORY	• To promote observational skills
MOTOR	• To develop fine motor skills
BEHAVIOUR	• To promote self-regulation of behaviour/impulsivity
EMOTIONS	• To promote group cohesion and trust
	• To promote a sense of ease and fun within the group

Top tips

○ Be aware of group members shouting out the answers. Explain why they should not shout out.

○ Objects could be selected around a theme (eg, school, transport or food).

○ Some group members may need help to remember the objects (writing lists, describing its function or appearance, drawing the objects, etc).

○ Be prepared to increase or decrease the number of objects as appropriate to the group.

○ This could be used as an introduction to a community visit (eg, things needed for a bus trip, things needed to make a pizza, options for eating out).

Routledge
Taylor & Francis Group
ROUTLEDGE

Activity levels

Level 1

- Place four objects on a flat surface and get the group to look at them.
- Pick up each object and name and describe it.
- Place the objects back on the flat surface and cover them with a cloth.
- Get the group to close their eyes or look away as you remove one of the objects.
- Ask one group member to identify which one is missing.
- Repeat until all group members have had a turn.

Level 2

- Gradually increase the number of objects.

Routledge
Taylor & Francis Group

Activity 18
Spot the differences

Equipment   None

Targets

LANGUAGE/ COMMUNICATION	• To develop inferencing skills • To promote expressive language
SOCIALISATION	• To develop 'Theory of Mind' (see Chapter 1)
SENSORY	• To promote observational skills
BEHAVIOUR	• To promote self-regulation of behaviour/impulsivity
EMOTIONS	• To create a sense of ease and fun within the group • To develop group cohesion and trust

Top tips

○ Some group members may not select a relevant difference for others to notice (eg, pulling socks up under trousers when no-one would be able to notice it). Always explain why this is not suitable and that it must be something the other group members can see.

○ Facilitators may need to model and further talk through this activity if the group are struggling.

○ Be wary of comments being too personal. If they are, explain why they are not positive things to say.

○ You can let the person who guessed correctly have the next turn, but be aware that some group members may never guess correctly. These individuals will need to be allowed a turn.

○ At Level 3, support may be needed to help group members to remember what the others looked like the week before. This could be done through drawings, written descriptions or photographs. This idea could even be carried into future groups and can prompt discussion about how we change (eg, hairstyles, fashions).

Routledge
Taylor & Francis Group

Activity levels

Level 1

- The group sit in a circle on the floor/chairs.
- One person is chosen. Explain that they will go out of the room with a group facilitator and change something about the way they look. Give examples, such as it may be their hairstyle or clothing.
- The chosen person goes into the centre of the circle and turns around so that every group member can see each detail of their appearance before something is altered. They then leave the room with a group facilitator.
- When outside the room, the group facilitator helps the individual to choose something to change about themselves (eg, take a shoe off, turn their jumper inside out).
- The group member and facilitator then return to the group.
- The individual stands in the middle of the circle again and turns around so that every group member can see them and try to identify what has changed.
- The group facilitators invite people with their hands up to guess what has changed.

Level 2

- The individual chooses what they want to change once outside the room more independently.
- The individual invites people with their hand up to guess what has changed.
- Fade out prompts from the group facilitators.

Level 3

- Group members examine and note the other group members' appearance. Encourage them to make notes or keep a record of this.
- The following week they discuss what is different from the week before (such as clothing or hairstyle). Some group members may need to refer back to their notes to facilitate this.

Routledge Taylor & Francis Group • **P** This page may be photocopied for instructional use only. *Groupwork for Children with ASD Ages 11–16* © A Eggett, K Old, LA Davidson & C Howe 2008

Activity 19
Mimes

Equipment   Cards with written word, line drawings or photographs of different actions and animals

Targets

LANGUAGE/ COMMUNICATION	• To develop sequencing skills (eg, sequence of gestures/ mimes)
	• To develop turn-taking
SOCIALISATION	• To develop creativity
	• To develop imagination
MOTOR	• To develop motor planning skills

Top tips

○ The group may need a high level of support as this is a skill that young people with ASD can find particularly difficult. For example, you may need to perform part or all of the mime and get them to copy it or perform alongside you. Some group members may need a verbal description of what to do. Some may need to be taken out of the room and allowed to practise the mime away from others before performing it in front of the group.

○ Be prepared to give prompts to help develop mimes if the rest of the group are finding it difficult to guess.

○ At Level 2, you may need to read what is on the card to group members with poor literacy skills. Take them out of the room to prevent other group members from overhearing.

○ If one or more group members are reluctant to put up their hand and guess, ensure that everyone suggests an action/animal after each mime. Start with different people if a group member is copying answers from others by going round all group members in turn.

○ At Level 3, encourage appropriate mimes as group members often pick a mime related to an obsession that others are not familiar with. Others may have something in mind that is impossible to mime, such as a specific model of train or a rare breed of shark. Discuss why the mime is difficult for others to guess and help to simplify it.

Routledge
Taylor & Francis Group
ROUTLEDGE

At Level 3, encourage longer sequences of mimes and relate them to a chosen theme (eg, using the bus to go bowling, or going to the cinema).

Activity levels

Level 1

Explain and model the activity to the group.

The group facilitator shows a card labelled with an action or animal to one group member.

The group member performs a mime to help the others guess what is on the card.

The others put their hands up to take turns in guessing.

Continue until everyone has had a turn.

Level 2

Each individual thinks of their own mime to perform. Some may need help to generate appropriate ideas.

Level 3

Select a theme that group members must relate their ideas to (eg, a community visit to the cinema).

Routledge
Taylor & Francis Group

Activity 20
Charades

Equipment   Small pieces of paper/card to write on (see the Activities card template in Appendix XIX for photocopiable blank cards to write on)

Targets

LANGUAGE/ COMMUNICATION	• To develop non-verbal communication skills • To improve interpretation of gesture
SOCIALISATION	• To promote teamwork skills
MOTOR	• To develop motor planning
EMOTIONS	• To explore emotional situations • To facilitate discussion of responses to emotive situations
SELF-AWARENESS AND COPING STRATEGIES	• To explore and promote appropriate coping strategies
INDEPENDENT LIVING	• To act out scenarios in a sequential order

Top tips

○ To begin with, use very easy topics and have a reserve of more difficult topics to move on to.

○ You can use scenarios that group members may find themselves in or use the activity as preparation for a community visit.

○ Be aware of motor planning issues that make miming very difficult.

○ The facilitator may have to support the group members who are guessing by directing attention to particular aspects of the mime.

Routledge
Taylor & Francis Group

P This page may be photocopied for instructional use only.

142

Activity levels

Level 1

- The group facilitators prepare cards labelled with well-known titles of books, television programmes, songs, etc.
- In turn, each group member picks a card and tries to convey the title by using non-verbal communication.
- Agree on common gestures to indicate cues (eg, 'sounds like' is indicated by pulling on your ear) and model these to the group.
- The person who guesses what is on the card then has a turn to choose a card and act out its contents.

Level 2

- The group can generate their own cards.

Level 3

- More emotive subjects and scenarios can be introduced, such as acting out emotions or being bullied.

Level 4

- The group can be split into two teams and do their mimes against the clock. Allow three minutes per turn, depending on the abilities of the group.
- Encourage team members to negotiate who will act out the idea to the other team.
- Encourage group members to negotiate how the winning team will be identified (eg, the first team to guess correctly three times).

Routledge
Taylor & Francis Group

Activity 21
Say the picture

 Equipment   Prepared game cards with words associated with your chosen theme (see the Activities card template in Appendix XIX for photocopiable blank cards to write on)
Pens/pencils

 Targets

LANGUAGE/ COMMUNICATION	• To develop the ability to interpret information and make predictions based on it • To develop recording skills – pictorial • To promote turn-taking
SOCIALISATION	• To develop awareness of others' appearance, personal characteristics and interests • To practise working as a team to achieve a desired result
LEISURE TIME AND INTERESTS	• To explore a range of interests and hobbies
EMOTIONS	• To develop group cohesion and trust • To explore a range of emotions
UNDERSTANDING OF DIAGNOSIS	• To promote awareness of their diagnosis

Top tips

○ Start with single words or concepts that can be communicated in a single picture.

○ Work towards more complex or elaborate ideas that may need to be communicated through a series of pictures.

Routledge
Taylor & Francis Group

Activity levels

Level 1

- Use a theme associated with issues that have been raised by individual group members (eg, bullying), group members' targets (eg, identifying emotions) or a forthcoming community visit (such as a trip to the bowling alley).
- Prepare a range of game cards in advance with different words related to the chosen theme.
- Each group member takes a turn to choose a game card and tries to communicate the word to the rest of the group using pictures.
- The other members of the group work together to try and guess what the individual is trying to communicate to them.

Level 2

- Encourage the group members to split into teams. Help them to negotiate how the group will be divided, which team will go first and the rules of the game (eg, the first team to get three answers right wins).
- Each team takes a turn. The team nominates a member to do the drawing for the other team to guess. Continue until one of the teams wins.

Level 3

- Encourage the group members to choose their own themes, identify associated words and, in teams, to prepare the game cards for the other team to guess.

Routledge
Taylor & Francis Group

Activity 22
Who am I?

Equipment   Stickers – enough for one per group member (and facilitators if they are joining in)
Pens
Headband
Cards

Targets

LANGUAGE/ COMMUNICATION	• To promote turn-taking • To develop the ability to ask and answer questions • To develop the use of closed questions
SOCIALISATION	• To promote staying on topic • To develop 'Theory of Mind' (see Chapter 1)
EMOTIONS	• To create a sense of ease and fun within the group • To create a sense of group trust

Top tips

○ Be aware of sensory issues when using stickers or a headband and do not insist if a group member feels uncomfortable with this.

○ Be aware of group interests and their knowledge base, for example, not all children are interested in soaps, pop stars, etc.

○ Be aware of obsessional interests at Level 2. Explain why someone may not be aware of the individual that they are thinking of.

○ The group may need some modelling of how to use closed questions.

○ You may want to limit the number of questions that one person asks to 20.

○ Prompt questions as needed (eg, 'Am I a boy?'). Some group members may need to repeat a question that you have given them.

○ Help the group to make links with regards to questions already asked. You may need to discuss information already gathered and why the new question is not appropriate.

○ Be prepared to give clues if someone is struggling.

Activity levels

Level 1

○ Before the group begins, select characters (eg, the Queen, a sports star, pop star, cartoon character) and write them on the stickers/headband.

○ Explain and model the activity.

○ Select one group member at a time, placing the sticker on their head/back/chair.

○ The individual with the sticker on asks one question at a time to try to find out who they are (eg, 'Am I male?').

○ The rest of the group can only answer with 'yes' or 'no'.

○ The individual continues to ask questions until they have guessed who they are.

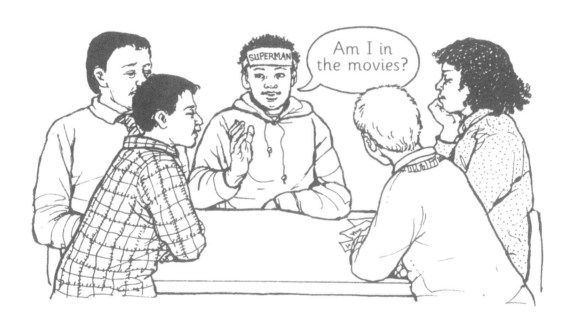

Level 2

○ One group member leaves the room while the rest of the group agree on a character for that group member. This encourages generation of ideas and provides opportunities for negotiation and compromise within the group.

Routledge
Taylor & Francis Group
ROUTLEDGE

Activity 23
Zoo

 Equipment   Chairs for each group member and facilitator except one

 Targets

LANGUAGE/ COMMUNICATION	• To develop vocabulary (eg, categories)
	• To develop auditory memory
	• To develop attention and listening skills
SOCIALISATION	• To learn group members' names
MOTOR	• To develop spatial awareness

 Top tips

○ It is important to consider safety. Make sure there is plenty of room for the activity.

○ Some group members will collide with each other. Think: is this a behaviour, motor planning or sensory issue?

○ Be aware of sensory overload. Some group members may require a calming activity after this (eg, five minutes 'chill-out' time).

○ If auditory defensiveness is an issue, try whispering names.

○ Be aware of motor planning issues for some young people. Encourage them to move around carefully to avoid collisions.

○ Some group members will struggle to think of zoo animals. You may need to give them clues or provide choices to help them to think of an animal, particularly if they are the last person to choose.

○ You may need a recap of animal names to begin with, to help group members to learn them.

○ When 'zoo' is called, make sure everyone swaps seats as some group members will try not to move.

○ You may need to demonstrate the activity a few times so that the group becomes familiar with it.

○ To expand vocabulary still further, play the game with the same rules but use different categories (eg, 'emotions', 'senses', 'worst lessons', 'favourite places').

Routledge
Taylor & Francis Group
ROUTLEDGE

Activity levels

Level 1

- Arrange enough seats in a wide circle for each group member and facilitator except one. The group facilitator without a chair stands in the middle of the circle.

- The group facilitator explains that she is an animal in the zoo and has lost her 'cage' (chair). She explains that all of the other animals (group members) have a 'cage' (chair) and she is going to try to get into one of their cages.

- The group facilitator chooses a zoo animal to be (eg, a penguin). The group members then each choose a different zoo animal to be (eg, a lion, snake or giraffe).

- The group facilitator explains that she will shout out the names of two animals who will swap places.

- As the animals swap places, the group facilitator tries to sit on one of their empty 'cages'.

- The person left in the middle then repeats the process.

- If a group member shouts out 'zoo' when they are in the middle, everyone must leave their 'cage' and find another.

Routledge
Taylor & Francis Group

Activity 24
Making sandwiches

Equipment   Plates for each group member
Knives
Bread suitable for sandwiches
Butter/margarine
Variety of sandwich fillings
Wipes/washing facilities

Targets

LANGUAGE/ COMMUNICATION	• To develop attention and listening skills • To develop requesting • To follow verbal instructions • To promote turn-taking • To develop vocabulary • To develop negotiation and compromise
SOCIALISATION	• To promote co-operative working • To promote sharing
SENSORY	• To develop sensory awareness (eg, tactile, proprioception, gustatory) • To develop awareness of own and others' personal space
MOTOR	• To promote fine motor skills • To develop bilateral skills • To develop hand–eye co-ordination
EMOTIONS	• To create a sense of ease and fun within the group • To create a sense of group trust • To identify and express a range of feelings

Routledge
Taylor & Francis Group
ROUTLEDGE

P

♡ Top tips

- Be sure to check out any allergies/dietary requirements.
- If a group member becomes anxious about mess, encourage him to wipe his hands and rejoin the activity.
- Encourage group members to share equipment and ingredients by reducing the amounts available. Model appropriate requesting if necessary.
- Some group members will need support to recall the sequence of the activity and the equipment needed. Encourage them to ask other group members for help.
- This is a good opportunity to talk about food preferences and differences within the group.
- At Level 2, refer to Shopping, Community visit G (see Chapter 8) before taking the group into the community.

Activity levels

Level 1

- Group members sit round a table.
- The group facilitator explains and models making a sandwich.
- Group members gather the equipment needed to make their sandwich.
- Group members make their own sandwiches.

Level 2

- Group members agree on a list of ingredients and go on a community visit to the shops to buy the ingredients for their sandwiches.

Routledge
Taylor & Francis Group

Activity 25
Treasure hunt

 Equipment   Treasure to hide (eg, puzzle, pencils, beanbag)
Blindfold (for Level 3)
Obstacles (for Level 4)

 Targets

LANGUAGE/ COMMUNICATION	• To follow verbal instructions • To develop problem-solving • To develop choice/decision-making
SOCIALISATION	• To promote and encourage teamwork • To develop negotiation and compromise • To consider others' views
LEISURE TIME AND INTERESTS	• To promote a wider experience of community activities
MOTOR	• To promote left/right orientation • To develop gross motor skills
INDEPENDENT LIVING	• To promote independent living skills in a community setting (eg, public transport, shop, café)
SELF-AWARENESS AND COPING STRATEGIES	• To promote confidence in accessing community experiences • To promote awareness of feelings of anxiety • To promote coping strategies in a community setting

Top tips

For all levels

○ This activity is best done regularly as it can be quite challenging and there are many levels to develop. This has the effect of promoting the group's self-confidence and sense of pride as they improve.

○ Be aware of sensory issues, especially vestibular processing difficulties, when blindfolded.

○ Model this activity to the group if necessary.

- Other group members should be encouraged to be quiet when it is not their turn.
- Use visual prompts to promote left/right orientation. A good way to learn this is to hold your hands up, palm facing away from you. This provides a natural capital 'L' on the left hand, using the index finger and the thumb, to signify 'left'. We have found this to be very helpful to group members when they are confused and we encourage them to look at this visual prompt when required.

For Levels 5 and 6

- Make sure members of the community involved in this activity are aware of what the task entails. Be aware of confidentiality issues.
- Be sensitive to group members' anxieties in an unfamiliar setting and with unfamiliar members of the public. Give positive reinforcement and explain what they have done well.
- Be aware of wider safety issues when out in the community and group members' anxieties relating to new experiences. Some pre-activity preparation is essential (eg, discussing bus timetables or what may happen on a treasure hunt) to help to reduce group members' anxiety.
- This activity requires careful pre-planning and risk assessment. Please refer to the section on community visits (see Chapter 8) for ideas and considerations around planning these.

Activity levels

Level 1

- One group member leaves the room.
- The group select a hiding place for the 'treasure'.
- The group member re-enters the room. The group facilitator directs the group member to the hidden treasure using simple instructions (eg, 'walk forward', 'stop', 'turn right'), until they reach the treasure.
- Continue until each group member has had a turn.

Level 2

- As Level 1, but group members take it in turn to give directions.

Level 3

- As above, but the group member finding the treasure is blindfolded to increase the challenge in finding the treasure.

Groupwork for Children with ASD Ages 11–16 © A Eggett, K Old, LA Davidson & C Howe 2008

Routledge
Taylor & Francis Group
ROUTLEDGE

Encourage the person giving directions to be more specific and give more feedback to facilitate the treasure seeker.

Level 4

- Add obstacles to negotiate.
- Again, encourage more specific directions and feedback to help the treasure seeker to negotiate these successfully.

Level 5

- Group facilitators design a treasure hunt around a small community setting (eg, the hospital or a school).
- Clues to finding the treasure are left with key members of this community (eg, the receptionist or canteen staff).
- The group and group facilitators follow the clues together to find the treasure.

Level 6

- Carry out the treasure hunt in a wider community setting, for example, clues could lead from the clinic via the bus to a café.

Routledge
Taylor & Francis Group

Activity 26
Token challenge

Equipment   Two rooms with a telephone in each
Pen and paper
Selection of activities /challenges
Tokens (eg, pictures of the reward)

Targets

LANGUAGE/ COMMUNICATION	• To develop attention and listening skills • To improve the ability to provide accurate information to others • To improve the ability to understand and follow verbal instructions
SOCIALISATION	• To promote teamwork skills • To promote consideration and awareness of others' strengths and needs • To develop and improve skills in negotiation, compromise and problem-solving
SENSORY	• To develop awareness and tolerance of individual sensory issues
MOTOR	• To improve motor co-ordination
EMOTIONS	• To develop confidence and self-esteem
INDEPENDENT LIVING	• To develop telephone skills

Top tips

At all levels, the group will need a high level of support to negotiate, compromise, reduce anxieties and encourage one another.

The group may need support in managing their time.

Have a wide variety of activities, including motor, sensory and cognitive tasks, for the challenges (eg, 'Pot five balls on the pool/snooker table within a set time (five minutes)', 'Throw five beanbags into/at a target within a set time (three minutes)', Charades, Hangman or the Feely bag game).

This page may be photocopied for instructional use only. *Groupwork for Children with ASD Ages 11–16* © A Eggett, K Old, LA Davidson & C Howe 2008

Routledge
Taylor & Francis Group

P

- At Level 3, dissuade from dangerous, unrealistic and unkind tasks. Discuss why.
- The tokens can lead to any reward that is meaningful for the group (eg, a choice of activities or school equipment).
- Activities such as Role plays (Activity 31) and Thought showers (Activity 33) are useful to develop telephone skills.
- When withdrawing individual group members to separate rooms, first consult local policies for child protection, health and safety and risk assessment.

Activity levels

Level 1

- Group facilitators explain the rules of the game.
- One group member goes with a facilitator into a separate room.
- The group facilitators pre-select an activity for each group member. This is written down and given to the individual for their turn.
- The group member then rejoins the group and informs the other group members of his task (eg, 'Pot five pool balls within four minutes').
- The group member has to complete the task and if successful will receive a token for the group.
- Each group member has a turn.
- At the end, there is a prize for the group if they reach a certain number of tokens.

Level 2

- One group member and group facilitator go into a different room.
- The remainder of the group stay in the main room.
- The group decide on a challenge for the individual group member with support from the group facilitator.
- The group negotiate who will telephone the individual group member and inform them of their challenge.
- The individual group member needs to answer the telephone, listen to the information and accept the challenge.
- The group are reunited whilst the group member carries out the challenge.
- Each group member has a turn.
- If the challenges are successfully completed, a token is received for the group.

Level 3

- The group is divided into two teams.
- The group devise their own challenges.
- The two teams take it in turn to telephone one another, describe and perform their challenges.

Routledge
Taylor & Francis Group

Activity 27
Group picnic game

Equipment   Ingredients to make a sandwich (eg, bread, butter, cheese/ ham)

Ingredients to ice biscuits (eg, biscuits, icing sugar, water, cake decorations)

Ingredients to make a fruit cocktail stick (eg, orange segments, grapes, banana, cocktail sticks)

Paper plates

Spoons, knives, bowls

Table and chairs/picnic rug

Targets

LANGUAGE/ COMMUNICATION	• To promote attention and listening skills • To promote turn-taking • To promote the ability to follow verbal and visual instructions • To promote the ability to give verbal and visual instructions
SOCIALISATION	• To promote teamwork skills • To develop skills of negotiation and compromise • To promote problem-solving skills
MOTOR	• To promote fine motor skills • To promote motor planning • To promote hand–eye co-ordination
EMOTIONS	• To create a sense of fun and ease within the group • To promote development and understanding of empathy
INDEPENDENT LIVING	• To promote and develop skills in basic food preparation • To promote budgeting skills • To promote and develop skills in going to the shops
SELF- AWARENESS AND COPING STRATEGIES	• To develop the ability to work in a small team • To identify and develop coping strategies to manage frustrations when working with others • To develop the ability to share these feelings with others

Routledge
Taylor & Francis Group

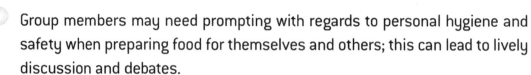

Top tips

- Group members may need prompting with regards to personal hygiene and safety when preparing food for themselves and others; this can lead to lively discussion and debates.
- Group members may need a lot of support to make the picnic items, from sequencing the activity to physically preparing the food items themselves. Be prepared to help in a supportive and encouraging way.
- Be aware of poor auditory memory. Some groups may need either written or visual instructions to guide them in this activity.
- Increase the number of tasks depending on the group members' abilities.
- Be sensitive to all group members and be aware of comments that group members may make; always discuss at the time why some are not appropriate.
- Encourage and promote discussion on becoming more independent, particularly in food preparation, budgeting and shopping.
- This activity often takes up the whole of the group activity time, so be aware of timing when planning.
- At Level 2, it is important that the facilitators carefully pre-select the pairs.
- At Levels 2 and 3, support may be required in helping the group members to work as a pair and in developing their skills in negotiation and compromise: always discuss why this is important.
- At Level 3, it is sometimes fun to add a timed element to the activity, thereby raising the level of challenge.
- If the group session is long enough, it is also beneficial for the group members to visit a shop to purchase the items needed prior to the activity taking place.

Activity levels

Level 1

- Provide each group member with space to work.
- The facilitators model making a sandwich, explaining to the group that they will have to do this next.
- Group members make their own sandwich.
- Facilitators model icing and decorating biscuits, explaining to the group that they will have to do this activity next.
- Group members ice and decorate their biscuits.
- Facilitators model making a fruit cocktail stick by putting a piece of banana, a grape and an orange segment onto the cocktail stick, explaining to the group that they will be doing this activity next.

Group members make their fruit cocktail stick.

All group members bring their food to a central point in the room (eg, lay a picnic rug on the floor or table) and participate in a group picnic.

Level 2

Explain to the group that they are going to play the Group picnic game.

Divide the group members up into pairs.

The group facilitator models making a sandwich, icing and decorating a biscuit and making a fruit cocktail stick.

Position the items where all the group members are able to see them.

The facilitator nominates one of each pair to make the sandwich and ice the biscuits and their partner must assist them with this.

Explain to the group that the third picnic item to be prepared must be negotiated between the pair themselves as to who makes, who assists or whether they share the role instead.

Group members make their items.

Group members share the food as a picnic.

Group members discuss their performance.

Level 3

The pairs decide which one of them will be in charge of making which items for the picnic.

Group members share their food and discuss their performance.

Routledge
Taylor & Francis Group

Activity 28
Good and bad things from the week

 Equipment   None

 Targets

LANGUAGE/ COMMUNICATION	• To practise making decisions and choices • To practise expressing information, feelings and opinions
EMOTIONS	• To promote group cohesion and trust
SELF-AWARENESS AND COPING STRATEGIES	• To explore and promote appropriate coping strategies in relation to situations of daily living and the emotions associated with them

 Top tips

○ Ensure that the group is able to deal sensitively with information shared. Consider any issues that you know have affected any individuals that may be difficult to disclose. For some groups, you may just focus on the positive if sensitive issues are not appropriate for group discussion.

○ If any issues are raised in the group that cause you concern (eg, any expression of self-harm, severe bullying, family issues or depression), then the appropriate professional and the individual's parent or carer need to be informed immediately.

○ You may need to give cues, examples and a limited choice of possible options to facilitate sharing of information, but everyone must try to say something.

○ Consider the suitability of advice. Point out if things are silly or dangerous.

○ Exchange email/phone numbers only if group members consent and group facilitators feel it is appropriate. Discussion about the social rules of telephone/ email etiquette needs to be raised.

Routledge
Taylor & Francis Group

Activity levels

Level 1

○ Take it in turn to say one positive thing that has happened during the week and one thing not so positive.

○ The group facilitator models appropriate responses to the information shared.

Level 2

○ Encourage group members to support each other. Share similar experiences, discuss and as a group try to identify appropriate responses and coping strategies.

Level 3

○ With a well-formed, gelled group, email/telephone numbers can be exchanged to encourage group members to keep in touch and discuss these issues outside the group.

Routledge
Taylor & Francis Group

Activity 29
Leaflets/questionnaires

Equipment　Paper
Pens
Word processor (optional)

Targets

LANGUAGE/ COMMUNICATION	• To develop turn-taking
	• To develop attention and listening skills
	• To develop expressive language
	• To develop the appropriate recording of information
SOCIALISATION	• To promote teamwork
	• To promote skills in compromise and negotiation
	• To promote the development of problem-solving skills
	• To consider others' viewpoints
SENSORY	• To increase awareness of sensory issues
MOTOR	• To increase awareness of motor issues
	• To promote fine motor skills
EMOTIONS	• To explore a range of emotions
	• To link emotions with real-life situations
INDEPENDENT LIVING	• To explore issues and feelings about independent living
UNDERSTANDING OF DIAGNOSIS	• To increase awareness and understanding of their diagnosis of ASD
	• To promote understanding of how their diagnosis impacts on themselves and others
SELF-AWARENESS AND COPING STRATEGIES	• To raise awareness of their own strengths and needs
	• To identify coping strategies in relation to themes important to them

Routledge
Taylor & Francis Group
ROUTLEDGE

TRANSITION	To explore issues and feelings around transitions (eg, diagnosis of ASD, moving schools)
	To problem-solve issues relating to transitions (eg, from secondary to further education)

Top tips

- Consider using a word processor to give a more professional finish. Typing is often an easier method of recording for some group members.
- You may need to break down the theme into more manageable areas (eg, a leaflet entitled 'Coping in school' could be divided into sections on bullying, lunchtimes, friendships).
- Facilitators will need to help with negotiation between group members.
- There will be a range of views and experiences and all of these need to be heard and managed in a sensitive way.
- The scribe may be best selected using fair means (eg, names from a hat or drawing numbers).
- This topic can lead to some lively debates which can lead into other themes that you may wish to explore in further sessions.
- This is an excellent debrief activity following a community visit.

Activity levels

Level 1

- Group facilitators agree on a theme that is appropriate for the group (eg, how to deal with bullies, hygiene, diagnosis, a community visit).
- Group facilitators explain to the group that they are going to design a leaflet or questionnaire.
- Group facilitators show examples of a leaflet/questionnaire to the group.
- The group members use a thought shower to determine the content of the leaflet/questionnaire (see Activity 33 for ideas).
- Group facilitators act as scribes, giving guidance as appropriate.

Level 2

- Group members negotiate a theme for the leaflet/questionnaire themselves.
- One group member is selected as the scribe.

Routledge
Taylor & Francis Group

Activity 30
Debates

Equipment   Video/television

Targets

LANGUAGE/ COMMUNICATION	• To develop turn-taking • To develop attention and listening skills • To develop expressive language skills relating to persuasion
SOCIALISATION	• To promote teamworking skills • To consider others' views • To promote skills in negotiation, compromise and problem-solving
EMOTIONS	• To explore a range of emotions • To increase awareness of their own and others' emotions
INDEPENDENT LIVING	• To explore and discuss issues relating to independent living
SELF-AWARENESS AND COPING STRATEGIES	• To promote and develop appropriate coping strategies
UNDERSTANDING OF DIAGNOSIS	• To promote awareness of diagnosis and how this relates to self and others
TRANSITIONS	• To explore and discuss issues relating to transitions

Top tips

- Set ground rules prior to debate (eg, no personal comments, no bad language).
- Be aware of high emotions, and the need to intervene and diffuse heated situations when they occur. Debrief group members and advise on coping strategies. Videoing is helpful with this.

Routledge
Taylor & Francis Group

- Some group members may find it difficult to assert themselves in the role of chair and will need support to carry this out.
- Set a time limit for the debate that is relevant to the ability and interests of group members. We have had debates last from five minutes to the whole session in length.
- Video the activity and reflect on elements of performance (eg, turn-taking, staying on topic).

Activity levels

Level 1

- The group facilitator chooses a topic for a debate (eg, bullying, school, friendships, fashion, personal hygiene, the need to develop independent living skills, understanding of diagnosis, transitions).
- Group facilitators explain and model the concept of a debate.
- A group facilitator divides the group members into 'for' and 'against' teams.
- A group facilitator takes on the role of chair.
- A debate is held.

Level 2

- Group members negotiate and select the topic.
- Group members put themselves into teams, using a fair method (eg, names from a hat, drawing numbers).
- Group members nominate a chair for the debate.

Groupwork for Children with ASD Ages 11–16 © A Eggett, K Old, LA Davidson & C Howe 2008

Routledge
Taylor & Francis Group
ROUTLEDGE

Activity 31
Role plays

 Equipment
Pre-planned scenarios and scripts
Video camera
Television with video player

 Targets

LANGUAGE/ COMMUNICATION	• To practise a range of conversational skills • To practise expressing information, feelings and opinions • To promote discussion and problem-solving
SOCIALISATION	• To promote friendship-making skills • To promote awareness of others' feelings, opinions and beliefs
LEISURE TIME	• To practise a range of activities of daily living and community skills
EMOTIONS	• To practise ways of expressing emotions appropriately
UNDERSTANDING OF DIAGNOSIS	• To promote awareness of their diagnosis and how to communicate this to others
SELF-AWARENESS AND COPING STRATEGIES	• To explore and promote appropriate coping strategies

 Top tips

○ Gain consent from parents, carers and the group members for videoing.

○ Some group members may need a high level of adult supervision to operate equipment. Be aware of any health and safety issues relating to the equipment being used.

○ A high level of one-to-one support may be needed for less able pairs.

○ Modelling and guided discussion is essential for this activity.

Routledge
Taylor & Francis Group

Model how to give feedback and be prepared to give lots of prompts.

At Level 4, some group members may need a specific target to look for when analysing themselves (eg, eye contact, turn-taking or observing body language). You may need to explain what these things are and why they are important for successful communication.

A room with a camera, recording facilities, television and video are needed for Levels 4 and 5.

Some group members may find being filmed anxiety provoking. This needs to be handled sensitively. A 'behind camera' role may be more suitable for these individuals until they are more relaxed and confident.

Activity levels

Level 1

Use a theme associated with issues that have been raised by individual group members (eg, bullying), group members' targets (eg, expressing emotions) or a forthcoming community visit (eg, a trip to the bowling alley).

Discuss scenarios that may arise with the group members. Explain that they are going to practise what they would say or do in these situations using role play.

Facilitators role play a chosen scenario. Encourage the group to talk about what was good about the facilitators' actions and what could be improved.

Put group members into ability-matched pairs.

Give each pair a script and encourage them to practise role playing the scenario.

Each pair takes a turn to act out their scenario to the group.

Group members then feed back what was good about the scripted scenario and what could be improved.

Level 2

Encourage the pairs to rewrite the script and change the words and actions appropriately to improve the scenario.

Level 3

Get the group members to generate their own scenarios and scripts without models or prompts.

Routledge
Taylor & Francis Group

Level 4

- Film the role plays.
- Get group members to watch back their role play in their pairs.
- Encourage them to reflect on their performance (eg, non-verbal communication, volume).

Level 5

- Group members not involved in the interview take on the role of operating the equipment, with each group member taking a turn. You may need to model this first. The pair engaging in the role play need to feel comfortable with being observed and commented on by other group members.

Routledge
Taylor & Francis Group

Activity 32
Quizzes

Equipment   Quiz sheets (see Appendix XXI for ideas of questions to use relating to ASD)
Pens/pencils

Targets

LANGUAGE/ COMMUNICATION	• To develop and improve turn-taking skills • To develop the ability to respond to questions
SOCIALISATION	• To promote teamwork skills • To promote and develop skills in negotiation, compromise and problem-solving
EMOTIONS	• To explore understanding of emotions
SELF-AWARENESS AND COPING STRATEGIES	• To explore appropriate coping strategies within daily life in relation to ASD • To understand others' reactions to behaviours
UNDERSTANDING OF DIAGNOSIS	• To explore individuals' understanding of ASD • To provide information on ASD
INDEPENDENT LIVING	• To raise awareness of activities of daily living, such as shopping and cooking • To develop understanding of budgeting skills
TRANSITIONS	• To explore issues that may be relevant to transitions, such as from secondary school to further education

Top tips

Initially, keep the quiz as a short introduction to or consolidation of another activity (eg, leaflets/questionnaires).

Use topical information for community visits (eg, prices of items in a supermarket prior to a shopping trip).

Differences of opinion can be used to develop a debate.

Routledge
Taylor & Francis Group
ROUTLEDGE

At Level 3, match pairs and be aware of any personality clashes. Group members may need support with negotiation.

The questions relating to ASD should be used with careful consideration to the group members. Only ask them if it is relevant to their targets, level of awareness, insight and acceptance of diagnosis of ASD.

Activity levels

Level 1

A group facilitator sets questions on a topic (eg, awareness of ASD).

Each group member has a quiz sheet and answers the questions independently.

A group facilitator then encourages group members to share their answers and leads a discussion on the chosen topic.

Level 2

As above, but the group members work in two teams and discuss the questions within the team prior to recording an answer. The group members need to negotiate their answers to the question.

A facilitator encourages the teams to share their answers, keeps scores and feeds back to the group.

Level 3

Group members split into pairs and design their own quiz questions to give to another pair/team.

Routledge
Taylor & Francis Group

Activity 33
Thought showers

Equipment   Pens
                  Paper

Targets

LANGUAGE/ COMMUNICATION	To develop receptive language skills To develop expressive language skills To develop attention and listening skills
SOCIALISATION	To develop and improve skills in negotiation, compromise and problem-solving To promote teamwork skills To promote awareness and consideration of others
LEISURE TIME AND INTERESTS	To identify and explore appropriate leisure pursuits and interests
SENSORY	To explore sensory issues relating to self
MOTOR	To explore issues relating to motor skills
EMOTIONS	To identify and explore a range of emotions
SELF- AWARENESS AND COPING STRATEGIES	To promote and develop self-awareness relating to a range of issues To promote and develop coping strategies to encourage independent living
UNDERSTANDING OF DIAGNOSIS	To promote awareness and understanding of their diagnosis of ASD
INDEPENDENT LIVING	To raise awareness of issues relating to independent living (eg, use of public transport, preparation of food, budgeting skills)
TRANSITIONS	To raise awareness of issues relating to transitions, such as from secondary to further education

Routledge
Taylor & Francis Group

Top tips

- A high level of support is required to promote negotiation and compromise.
- Topics can become highly emotive and support may be required to calm strong feelings.
- Pick a scribe carefully at Levels 2 and 3. It may give an opportunity for less vocal members to have a role. Dominant group members should not be scribes in case they take over the activity.

Activity levels

Level 1

- Group facilitators explain the activity to the group.
- One group facilitator acts as a scribe.
- The group facilitator selects the topic for discussion (eg, diagnosis, bullying, shopping).
- Group members volunteer thoughts, ideas and beliefs relating to the topic.
- The group facilitator writes them on the piece of paper.

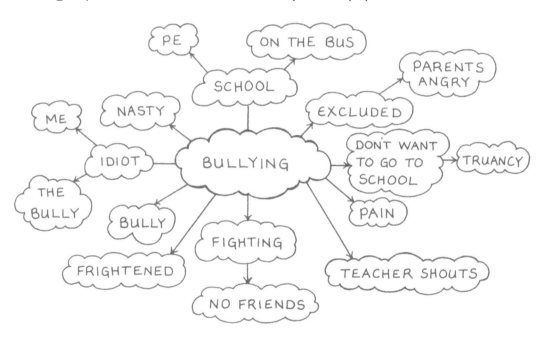

Level 2

- The group members negotiate a topic to discuss with support from the group facilitator.
- The group selects a scribe.

Level 3

- Group members complete the activity independently and feed back their ideas to the group facilitators.

Activity 34
Act out emotions

Equipment Prepared game cards with words associated with feelings/ emotions (see the Activities card template in Appendix XIX for photocopiable blank cards to write on)

Targets

LANGUAGE/ COMMUNICATION	• To develop understanding of feelings and emotions • To practise expressing feelings and emotions • To facilitate discussion about responses to emotive situations
SOCIALISATION	• To increase awareness of similarities and differences with peers • To promote teamwork skills
EMOTIONS	• To develop group cohesion and trust • To explore emotional situations and identify appropriate coping strategies to manage these
UNDERSTANDING OF DIAGNOSIS	• To promote awareness of their diagnosis of ASD

Top tips

- Group members may have some difficulties in understanding abstract concepts. Use visual helpers and explain concepts fully to develop their understanding.
- Be aware of emotive issues that may come up. Group members may require high levels of support when exploring emotive issues.
- Allow time out of the activity if required.
- Levels 2 and 3 are best used when the group is well-established.
- Use this activity to explore feelings about ASD – the group members could choose to act out words related to how they feel about their diagnosis.

Routledge
Taylor & Francis Group

Activity levels

Level 1

○ Prepare cards in advance with different words associated with feelings and emotions (eg, 'happy', 'angry', 'surprised').

○ One group member chooses a card and tries to communicate the word to the rest of the group using gestures/mime.

○ The group member then passes the turn on to the next person who also tries to communicate a word using a different gesture/mime.

○ Continue passing the turn on until each group member has tried to express a word in gestures/mimes in their own way.

○ Each group member takes a turn to choose a card and start the activity.

Level 2

○ Encourage the group members to think of their own words relating to feelings and emotions to pass around the group.

○ Encourage the group members to think about a situation in which they experienced that feeling or emotion and share it with the group during their turn.

Level 3

○ Encourage the group members to discuss how they reacted in that situation.

○ Encourage the group members to think of other things that they could say or do in such a situation.

Routledge
Taylor & Francis Group
ROUTLEDGE
P

Activity 35
Planets

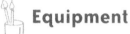

Equipment　　Circles of different size, colour and texture
Card and collage materials (see Appendix VII)
Large pieces of black paper

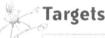

Targets

LANGUAGE/ COMMUNICATION	• To develop the ability to ask and answer questions
	• To develop negotiation skills
	• To develop understanding of abstract concepts
	• To develop listening and attention skills
	• To practise expressing information, feelings and opinions
SOCIALISATION	• To develop self-awareness
	• To develop awareness of others
EMOTIONS	• To explore the meaning of close relationships
	• To facilitate the expression of feelings about interpersonal relationships
SELF-AWARENESS AND COPING STRATEGIES	• To develop awareness of how individuals are seen by others
	• To explore differences in closeness at different times

Top tips

Many group members will struggle with the concept of somebody being 'close' to them. Some group members may take it literally (eg, someone sitting in close proximity to them). Therefore, you may need to explore this concept prior to carrying out the activity.

Be prepared to give some group members one-to-one attention during this activity.

The group members can include pets and friends on their list as well as family.

Some group members will want to be precise and use rulers, numbers and percentages to be accurate; this is fine.

This page may be photocopied for instructional use only. *Groupwork for Children with ASD Ages 11–16* © A Eggett, K Old, LA Davidson & C Howe 2008

Routledge
Taylor & Francis Group

P

- This activity could be done on the computer if the group members are more motivated to do this.
- Encourage group members to listen and be supportive to others' feedback regarding their own relationships.
- At Level 3, it is important that the group is well established and that all group members are listened to and supported.

Activity levels

Level 1

- Give each group member a piece of black paper and a selection of circles.
- Explain that they are going to make a picture of their universe, using the circles to represent people in their life.
- Get them to write down a list of the people who are most important in their life.
- Ask group members to choose a circle for each person and write their name on the circle.
- Ask them to choose a circle for themselves and stick it in the middle of the paper.
- Talk to the group about people we feel close to and people we do not.
- Let them place the rest of the circles on the paper surrounding their circle according to how close they feel they are to them.
- Ask each group member to share their picture with the group in turn.

Level 2

- Use the concept of the circles being planets in the universe.
- Ask group members to create a planet first for themselves and then for the other people in their life.
- Support them in identifying characteristics in others and ways to represent this (eg, using different sizes, colours and textures).
- Ask each group member to share their universe with the group.

Level 3

- Use only one piece of paper.
- Each group member has a planet to make of their own.
- They then discuss how and where each of their planets are placed on the paper according to the group dynamics.
- The group members could also be asked to make a planet for another individual in the group.

Routledge
Taylor & Francis Group
ROUTLEDGE

Activity 36
Emotional thermometers

Equipment   Large piece of paper
Coloured pens
Emotional thermometer template (see Appendix XXIII)

Targets

LANGUAGE/ COMMUNICATION	• To increase understanding of vocabulary relating to feelings and emotions • To develop expression of feelings and emotions • To facilitate discussion and responses to emotive situations
SOCIALISATION	• To share experiences with group members
EMOTIONS	• To explore and identify a range of emotions • To develop awareness of emotional extremes (eg, happy, sad, angry, calm)
SELF-AWARENESS AND COPING STRATEGIES	• To understand emotional reactions to different situations (eg, shouting, crying, physical confrontation, walking away) • To explore behavioural, cognitive and physical coping strategies to manage difficult emotions and situations
INDEPENDENT LIVING	• To link emotions with real-life situations and explore how they impact on independent living

Top tips

Group members may have some difficulties in understanding abstract concepts. Therefore a high level of support may be needed.

Be aware that some issues may be sensitive and need careful management and support.

This activity is best used when the group is well-established.

Prior to carrying out Level 2, it is useful to hold a discussion about good and not so good ways to handle difficult emotions and appropriate coping strategies.

This page may be photocopied for instructional use only. *Groupwork for Children with ASD Ages 11–16* © A Eggett, K Old, LA Davidson & C Howe 2008

Routledge
Taylor & Francis Group

Activity levels

Level 1

○ Group facilitators explain the activity to the group.

○ Each group member is given a sheet of paper and draws a thermometer the length of the paper. The thermometers are marked at regular intervals. Alternatively, group members could use the emotional thermometer template provided in Appendix XXIII.

○ The group facilitator chooses an emotion, such as 'anger'.

○ The group members think of different ways in which they experience this emotion and grade them using the emotional thermometer.

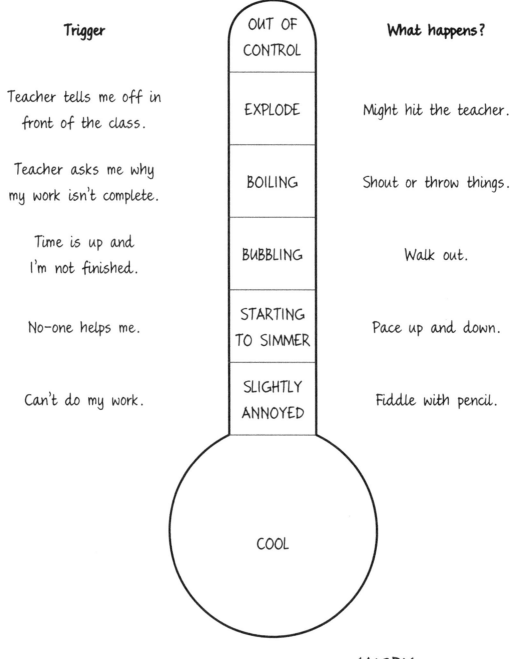

Trigger		What happens?
	OUT OF CONTROL	
Teacher tells me off in front of the class.	EXPLODE	Might hit the teacher.
Teacher asks me why my work isn't complete.	BOILING	Shout or throw things.
Time is up and I'm not finished.	BUBBLING	Walk out.
No-one helps me.	STARTING TO SIMMER	Pace up and down.
Can't do my work.	SLIGHTLY ANNOYED	Fiddle with pencil.
	COOL	

The feeling we are describing is _____ANGRY_____

Each group member thinks of situations where they felt this emotion. The situations may also be plotted on the thermometer, alongside the appropriate description of how they would feel in that situation.

Triggers and behavioural responses may also be useful information to add on.

The group members take it in turn to share their personal thermometer with the group.

Level 2

When the emotions, triggers and behaviour are plotted, the individual can start to think about coping strategies in each of the situations.

Physical symptoms (such as a red face, headache, sore tummy) can also be discussed to help individuals to recognise their emotional state.

Discuss colours and how they link with emotions (eg, envy – green, anger – red). These can be plotted on their thermometer if desired.

A small version can be made, for example, one small enough to make into a key ring and carry with them to use as a prompt in everyday situations.

Routledge
Taylor & Francis Group

Activity 37
Life maps

 Equipment   Large pieces of paper
Coloured pens

 Targets

LANGUAGE/ COMMUNICATION	• To develop expression of feelings and emotions • To develop attention and listening skills • To discuss responses to emotive situations and life events
SOCIALISATION	• To share experiences with group members
EMOTIONS	• To link thoughts to feelings and actions
SELF- AWARENESS AND COPING STRATEGIES	• To develop self-awareness • To promote development of appropriate coping strategies
AWARENESS OF DIAGNOSIS	• To explore feelings from around the time of being given a diagnosis of ASD • To promote the externalisation of thought processes about these feelings
INDEPENDENT LIVING	• To explore realistic goals for the future • To identify areas of need within independent living
TRANSITIONS	• To identify times that may cause difficulty, such as moving from secondary to further education • To assist in planning for the future (eg, goal setting, career options)

 Top tips

Group facilitators need to be aware of any sensitive issues raised within the group (eg, bereavements, issues around diagnosis) and support will need to be put into place to manage this. Consider referral to outside agencies if appropriate and consent is given.

Routledge
Taylor & Francis Group

Allow the group members to feed back as much or as little as they feel comfortable with; there may be some very sensitive information to share.

Some group members may need a high level of support during this activity.

If necessary, give suggestions of things that they might include as some people have problems creating ideas.

Help with writing may be necessary. Explore alternative methods of recording (eg, using the computer, drawing).

Activity levels

Level 1

Group facilitators explain the activity to the group members.

Each group member is given a piece of paper.

Each group member draws a road, starting at the left-hand side of the paper and ending at the right-hand side.

The group facilitator demonstrates placing on the road significant things that have happened to them over their life (eg, the birth of siblings, house moves, taking up hobbies, deaths, school transitions).

Each group member completes their life map.

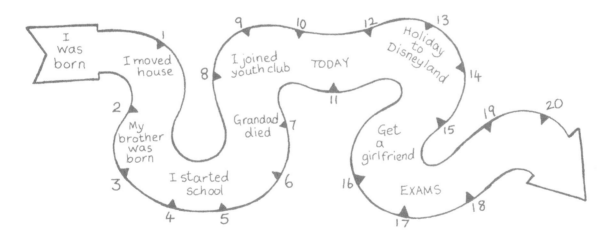

They are asked to circle in a favourite colour all of the good times and use a different colour to highlight all of the bad times.

The group members take it in turn to share their map with the rest of the group.

Level 2

Create another road to represent the future.

Choose what time-frame to work on (eg, five years, twenty years).

The group members think about the next few years, what they want to achieve and how they are going to do this.

P This page may be photocopied for instructional use only. *Groupwork for Children with ASD Ages 11–16* © A Eggett, K Old, LA Davidson & C Howe 2008

Routledge
Taylor & Francis Group

Activity 38
Power circles

 Equipment
Large card circle with a dot in the middle
10–30 blank cards
Glue
Pens/pencils

 Targets

LANGUAGE/ COMMUNICATION	• To encourage expression of ideas, thoughts and feelings • To develop and improve skills in negotiation and compromise
SOCIALISATION	• To explore role boundaries (eg, adult/child; teacher/ student) • To develop social awareness
EMOTIONS	• To facilitate expression of feelings about interpersonal relationships

 Top tips

○ You will have to explain what you mean by 'power', as some group members will take it literally. This could be a topic for discussion prior to engaging in the activity.

○ This can be an emotive activity and is best carried out in a well-established group with a good understanding of the issues that may arise.

○ There may be personal issues and experiences that will need to be sensitively handled throughout the session (eg, bullying, diagnosis). Consider referral to outside agencies if appropriate and consented to.

○ Group members may need a high level of support to negotiate, compromise and listen to others' thoughts and opinions.

Routledge
Taylor & Francis Group

Activity levels

Level 1

- Place the large circle of card on a table in the middle of the group.
- Explain that this is a circle of power and that the most powerful place is in the middle on the dot. The further out you go the less power you have.
- Have a selection of cards already written with common generic names on (such as 'teacher', 'police officer', 'bully', 'fire person', 'soldier', 'queen', 'baby').
- Give each group member a number of cards to place on the circle.
- Each group member has a turn at positioning their card on the circle and explains why they think that individual has that level of power.

Level 2

- The group members are asked to come up with other people who should be included in the circle (eg, family member, teacher, coach).
- The group members make a card for themselves.
- They may add their card and the other people they know to the power circle and address personal issues about power imbalances in discussion with the group (eg, the perception of the 'team leader' having more authority than other group members or of the victim having less power than the bully).
- Discuss good and bad power.
- Discuss how the group members make themselves more or less powerful and for what reasons.

Routledge
Taylor & Francis Group

Activity 39
The colour of feelings

 Equipment   Large pieces of paper
Paint
Brushes, sponges, string, to paint with, etc

 Targets

LANGUAGE/ COMMUNICATION	• To encourage the expression of feelings and emotions
SOCIALISATION	• To develop and improve skills in negotiation, compromise and problem-solving • To develop and promote teamwork skills
EMOTIONS	• To explore and identify a range of emotions • To link thoughts to feelings and actions • To promote the externalisation of thought processes

 Top tips

For all levels

○ Be aware of sensory issues to do with paint on hands, clothes, etc. Allow the use of utensils and for hands to be washed to decrease the level of distress.

○ Allow the individual group members to contribute as much or as little as they feel comfortable with.

○ Due to the inherent difficulties with abstract concepts for some group members, the symbolic nature of this activity may be hard for them to understand. It is still a good activity to help them to explore how feelings interact.

○ Some group members may need a high level of support during this activity.

For Level 3

The group picture can be used to decorate the group room of your chosen venue. This could be added to each week and can be referred to during other activity discussions to help the young people to understand their emotions.

Support will be needed to promote negotiation and compromise amongst the group members.

Activity levels

Level 1

The group facilitator explains the activity to the group.

Each group member has a piece of paper.

They are asked to write down all the feelings that they know about.

Each group member reads out their list to the group. The group facilitator encourages discussion of each feeling as it is read out.

Each group member grades the feelings on their list from most positive to most negative.

Each feeling is assigned a colour by the individual.

The colours associated with the feelings are painted in lines across a piece of paper from top to bottom going from positive at the top to negative at the bottom.

The group members then share their picture with the group.

Level 2

Encourage more abstract representations of the feelings (eg, rather than lines, group members may use swirling patterns or different textures).

Use two colours together to represent mixed feelings.

Level 3

Use rolls of wallpaper to make a large floor painting.

The group members all work together to create a large painting about feelings.

Routledge
Taylor & Francis Group

Activity 40
What's in my head?

Equipment

Picture of the brain (see Appendix XXII)
Coloured pens

Targets

LANGUAGE/ COMMUNICATION	• To encourage expression of thoughts, feelings and emotions
EMOTIONS	• To identify a range of emotions • To link thoughts to feelings and actions
SELF-AWARENESS AND COPING STRATEGIES	• To develop self-awareness • To promote development of appropriate coping strategies within daily living

Top tips

○ This can be an emotive activity, during which a number of sensitive issues may arise, and is therefore best carried out in a well-established group. Onward referral to outside agencies may be appropriate; consent will be required for this.

○ Some group members may require a high level of support during this activity.

○ This provides opportunities for discussion about sayings related to the brain (eg, 'It's at the back of my mind').

Activity levels

Level 1

○ The group facilitators explain the activity to the group.

○ Each group member has a picture of a head with a brain.

○ They are asked to write down the ten most common things that they think about (eg, school, friendships/relationships, hobbies/interests).

- Each topic should then be given a percentage or a mark out of ten according to how much they think about it.
- The brain picture is split into the number of topics discussed and each topic is allocated a proportion of the brain commensurate with its percentage or mark out of ten.
- Each topic is written in the appropriate section of the brain.
- Topics/thoughts can be colour-coded if appropriate (eg, happy thoughts – yellow).
- Each group member presents their 'brain' to the rest of the group.

Level 2

- Each group member completes their own picture. Before sharing them with the group, each individual is asked to guess what one of the other group members may have on their picture.

Level 3

- If a group member is bothered by recurring thoughts or worries, these can be described as being at the front of their mind. The group can discuss ways to help put these thoughts further back (eg, try to put other thoughts in their place).
- Group members are asked to link thoughts to actions and either write or draw what they do when they have a thought.

This has been adapted from an original activity. Written by Margot Sunderland and illustrated by Philip Engleheart, 1993. *Draw on Your Emotions: Creative Ways to Explore, Express and Understand Important Feelings*, Speechmark Publishing, Milton Keynes.

Routledge
Taylor & Francis Group

Community visits

ommunity visits are used to develop and transfer skills learned in the group sessions into 'real-life' situations. All of the skills targeted in the group sessions are intended to be functional and generalised into everyday settings. The community visits act as a 'stepping stone' to facilitate generalisation of skills from the group sessions through a supported community activity before becoming fully independent.

How to use the community visits

For the purpose of this book, we have chosen a sample of the community visits that we have successfully carried out with groups in our local community. These are by no means exhaustive, and you may have your own ideas for possible community visits, depending on your group members' needs and also the resources and funding that you have available when planning. The practicalities of carrying out our suggested community visits will depend on the area that you work in and the facilities available within your area. Our service is located on the coast and we therefore have easy access to the beach, but we are aware that this is an activity that will not be practical for a number of groups.

The community visits have been divided into the two different levels referred to elsewhere in the book: the *emerging independence* stage (11–13 years) and the *facilitating independence* stage (14–16 years). The levels and corresponding ages should be used with care, discretion and flexibility. For example, in one group you may have some group members following targets at the emerging independence stage and some at the facilitating independence stage depending on their availability levels and prior experience of groupwork.

Community visits at the emerging independence stage focus on carrying out activities that develop prerequisite skills that young people need in order to become more independent within everyday activities and the community. At the facilitating independence stage, the emphasis is placed on group members planning and carrying out community visits as independently as possible. Support from group facilitators is still required at this level, but greater autonomy is given to group members.

For community visits to be a success, it is essential that you have planned and are well-prepared, that all necessary risk assessments have been carried out and that consent has been obtained prior to the visit taking place. For this reason, it is important to read the Top tips provided.

All of the visits can be carried out within a timeframe of 90 minutes to two hours and have proved popular with our group members.

○ General information about the visits

Planning community visits

The number and timing of community visits within the groupwork timetable will vary, dependent on the skills and needs of your individual group members. For example, the timetable for a group consisting of young people who have not met before or a group with a high proportion of group members at the emerging independence stage may include just one community visit. The same may be true if the group includes a number of members raising specific issues (eg, concerns about bullying). In these situations the community visit may take place towards the end of the group when the young people have got to know each better, have had opportunities to practise the skills required to make the visit successful in the safety of the group setting or when other issues have been dealt with.

On the other hand, a well-established group with a high proportion of young people at the facilitating independence stage may include several community visits on their timetable that take place throughout the group, allowing time to plan and debrief in between them. For these young people, the emphasis is on getting out into the community and developing their independence skills and confidence, rather than being in the clinic or school setting.

Equipment

See the description of each visit for details of any equipment required.

Targets

All of the community visits in this chapter have the following general aims:

- To increase awareness of the skills required within the young person's identified target areas
- To practise emerging skills with support in everyday situations
- To use skills with increasing independence in everyday situations

These targets may be applied to any of the areas of need listed below:

- Language and communication skills
- Socialisation
- Leisure time and interests
- Sensory issues
- Motor skills
- Behaviour
- Emotional development

○ Understanding of diagnosis
○ Transitions
○ Self-awareness and coping strategies
○ Independent living skills

Top tips

○ Ensure that risk assessment forms have been completed for the young people and the environment prior to each community visit being carried out.

○ Ensure that parents and carers are fully aware of what the community visit entails and that consent is given.

○ A higher staff ratio may be needed for some community visits. Staffing levels are determined by the type of visit and the abilities of the group members. Refer to your organisation's policies on staffing levels.

○ Many activities will incur a cost. We have negotiated with our management a budget that we are able to spend on each community visit. Bear in mind that the cost of visits may be prohibitive for some group members if they are required to pay themselves.

○ Budgets should be explained to the group members in the planning sessions before the community visit. This helps to develop their planning and negotiation skills, avoids confusion and increases their awareness of others. For example, it might be inappropriate to bring a lot of extra spending money on a trip if it makes some of the group members feel uncomfortable.

○ Following a community visit, debriefing is essential. This gives group members the opportunity to express their feelings associated with the visit, and to say what went well and what did not. Problem-solving around any issues raised can then take place. Activities such as Friendship darts (Activity 6), Pool (Activity 9), Leaflets/questionnaires (Activity 29), Role plays (Activity 31), and Thought showers (Activity 33) are useful for this. Videoing community visits to analyse and discuss issues within the group can also be useful. Consent should be gained from parents, carers and the group members themselves before video recording.

○ Ensure that you know your group members with regard to what behaviours they may display and what triggers these behaviours. Some community visits may not be suitable (eg, a beach trip where one group member has a tendency to run off).

○ To use community visits effectively, we would recommend that you need one session for preparation activities, one for the community visit itself and one for debriefing. This can be altered, depending upon the needs of the group (eg, increase the number of preparatory sessions).

A wordsearch (an example is provided in Appendix XXVI) can be created to help group members generate ideas for where they want to go. Further wordsearches based on the chosen visit can be created to raise awareness of important things, for example, one based on swimming may include vocabulary such as 'towel', 'changing rooms' and 'lockers'.

Emerging independence stage

At the emerging independence stage, preparation activities must be carried out in the session before the community visit takes place. This helps group members to prepare and practise the skills required for the visit before they are incorporated into a real-life situation. Always explain how the activity links with the skill required, for example, Token challenge (Activity 26) with phoning for a pizza and Thought showers (Activity 33) with identifying ingredients for a pizza or writing a shopping list.

The following activities are all very versatile and therefore good in developing the prerequisite skills at this stage:

- Role plays (Activity 31) help to practise specific skills (eg, asking for food).
- Zoo (Activity 23) can teach the basic skills needed for team games.
- Friendship darts (Activity 6), Hangman (Activity 12), Kim's game (Activity 17), Charades (Activity 20) and Say the picture (Activity 21) can all be played with a specific theme, relevant to one of the visits.
- Friendship darts (Activity 6) and Leaflets/questionnaires (Activity 29) are useful debriefing activities.
- Themed wordsearches. See Appendix XXVI for an example. You can create your own wordsearches for specific topics using the following website: www.puzzlemaker. school.discovery.com/WordSearchSetupForm.html
- Thought showers (Activity 33) are helpful for planning and preparing group members for their outing. They could focus on topics such as what the group may see at the beach or what they need to take.

Carry out the chosen community activity with agreed levels of support.

Facilitating independence stage

Group members should be encouraged to plan and carry out community visits as independently as possible. The level of group facilitator involvement is determined by the activity (eg, the facilitators' presence is required for community visits but would not be required if group members planned visits to each other's houses with the consent of parents or carers) and the skill mix and personalities of the group members. Activities to develop prerequisite skills (as above) may still be beneficial at this stage.

At this stage, different levels of support may be needed for the individual group members. For example, some group members may be competent at using the bus, whereas others will need help in asking the driver for a ticket or with organising their money. Your assessment and the group member's performance at the emerging independence stage should inform the levels of support provided. It may be appropriate to encourage group members to support each other rather than providing group facilitators to support them.

◉ List of community visits

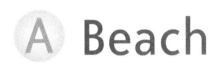 A Beach

 Equipment   Equipment for team games (eg, football, cricket)
Funding if having a snack or using public transport

Top tips

- Supervision and safety is a priority as the beach is an open area with many potential dangers. The staffing ratio may need to be higher because of the unstructured nature of the activity.
- Be aware of sensory issues (eg, tactile sensitivity to sand).
- The beach provides opportunities to carry out a range of activities (team games, sport, collecting items for Show and tell (Activity 4), buying snacks).
- If you are going to buy food or drink, see also Café (Community visit B).

Independence levels

Emerging independence

Further activities to develop prerequisite skills include:

- Snack time, where members take on different roles (eg, placing orders) or Role play (Activity 31) to practise scenarios associated with buying food or drink.
- Knowing your preferences (Activity 11) could be used to explore sensory issues (eg, sensitivity to textures on bare feet).

Group members may need support in the following aspects of this activity:

- Participating in team games.
- Identifying when they are over-stimulated and using calming strategies.

Facilitating independence

- Introduce Public transport (Community visit F) where possible.

This page may be photocopied for instructional use only. *Groupwork for Children with ASD Ages 11–16* © A Eggett, K Old, LA Davidson & C Howe 2008

Routledge
Taylor & Francis Group

B Café

Groupwork for Children with ASD Ages 11–16 © A Eggett, K Old, LA Davidson & C Howe 2008

Equipment   Funding for a snack and public transport, if required

Top tips

- Consider any allergies or dietary issues that may be relevant.
- Be aware of sensory issues (eg, taste, texture, noise, smell) and how these affect group members.
- At both levels, support may be needed to help group members to negotiate.
- Consider the time of your visit; you may want to avoid peak times.
- Set a designated meeting point.
- A high staffing ratio may be required, depending on your group members' needs and abilities.

Independence levels

Emerging independence

Further activities to develop prerequisite skills include:

- Snack time, where members take on different roles (eg, a waiter), can provide opportunities to do role plays (Activity 31) to rehearse likely scenarios.
- Knowing your preferences (Activity 11) could help to identify any oral sensitivity issues.

Group members may need support in the following aspects of this activity:

- Being aware of food tolerance and sensory preferences.
- Anxiety about eating in company.

Facilitating independence

- Group members negotiate where to go.
- Group members are given a budget and asked to stick to it. A group budget will add the need for negotiation and compromise.
- Group members are encouraged to pay and get a receipt for their own snack.
- Introduce Public transport (Community visit F) where possible.

Routledge
Taylor & Francis Group
ROUTLEDGE

C Cinema

Equipment   Funding for the visit (including transport, entrance fee and snacks)

Top tips

Consider supervision and safety. The cinema may be busy with many different areas to visit. Agree in advance whether you will stay together or whether different group members may do different things (eg, going to a café, playing computer games). Depending on this, the staffing ratio may need to be higher.

Check in advance when suitable films will be showing to ensure that you are going on the appropriate date and at the appropriate time.

Agree which film you want to see and what to do if there is a problem (eg, the film is sold out) in advance.

If you are going to buy food or drink, see also Café (Community visit B).

Independence levels

Emerging independence

Group members may need support in the following aspects of this activity:

Using the telephone or leaflets to find out film dates and times

Buying the tickets

Choosing and ordering snacks

Taking turns (eg, on computer games)

Coping with sensory issues (eg, noise, lighting, proximity to others)

Facilitating independence

Introduce Public transport (Community visit F) where possible.

Routledge
Taylor & Francis Group

D Going for a pizza

Equipment   Funding for the visit (including transport and food)

Top tips

- Check any allergies or dietary needs and help the group member to identify appropriate choices on the menu.
- Be aware of any food tolerance and sensory issues (eg, noise, lighting, smells).
- At both levels, support will be required to help negotiation and compromise.
- Look at a copy of the menu in group sessions prior to your visit to familiarise group members with the choices and layout.
- Discuss in advance whether the group would like starters, main course and/or dessert. Prepare them for people's different preferences and the possibility of waiting whilst others complete their meal.

Independence levels

Emerging independence

Further activities to develop prerequisite skills include:

- Cookery activities and snack time within the group sessions – these give a chance to observe group members' eating and drinking skills (eg, using a knife and fork), food preferences and sensory issues and choice/decision-making skills.
- Role plays (Activity 31) help to practise specific skills (eg, ordering from the menu).
- Knowing your preferences (Activity 11) is a useful activity for identifying any sensory issues and in providing coping strategies to manage these within such an environment.

Group members may need support in the following aspects of this activity:

- Making a reservation
- Informing the restaurant of the booking on arrival
- Reading from the menu
- Making choices/decisions
- Taking turns to order
- Ordering food and drinks
- Coping with sensory issues (eg, noise, lighting, movements, proximity to others, taste and texture)
- Asking for the bill

Facilitating independence

- Encourage group members to consider issues such as budgeting and to pay the bill independently to practise money skills.
- Introduce Public transport (Community visit F) where possible.

Routledge
Taylor & Francis Group

E Laser quest

This page may be photocopied for instructional use only. Groupwork for Children with ASD Ages 11–16 © A Eggett, K Old, LA Davidson & C Howe 2008

 Equipment   Funding for the session (including any transport and food)

 Top tips

- Be aware of any sensory issues (eg, noise, touch, movement, flashing lights, people).
- At both stages, support may be needed to help negotiation and compromise.
- Be supportive to group members who may display anxieties about being in such an environment.
- Consider times of visits in order to avoid or be prepared for busy periods.
- The group members should all meet at a designated point.
- It may be useful to work out a timetable for the visit including travel times.

 Independence levels

Emerging independence

Further activities to develop prerequisite skills include:

- Knowing your preferences (Activity 11) is helpful to look at reactions (eg, to dark, vibration, smell).
- An obstacle course (Activity 15) to practise negotiating apparatus in dim light may be helpful in identifying potential difficulties.
- Token challenge (Activity 26) can be used to rehearse telephone skills and practise motor activities.

Group members may need support in the following aspects of this activity:

- Fear of the dark
- Disorientation
- Sensory overload

Facilitating independence

- Group members are asked to take control of paying admission fees and for refreshments, thus looking at budgeting skills.
- Introduce Public transport (Community visit F) where possible.
- Group members are responsible for checking and booking times.
- Group members are encouraged to be responsible for negotiating teams and rules, with support when necessary.

Routledge
Taylor & Francis Group
ROUTLEDGE

F Public transport

Equipment   Timetables/maps
                 Funding

Top tips

- Be aware of any sensory issues (eg, travel sickness, close proximity to others, noise).
- At the facilitating independence stage, it may be useful for group members to observe aspects of this activity first (such as recording information during a telephone call).
- Consider transport times and how they fit in with other community visits (eg, restaurant bookings, film starting times).
- Check travel times and whether the route goes directly to your destination. Consider how long it will take to complete the journey and whether more than one mode of transport is required.
- Be aware of the complexity of the journey – start by using only one mode of transport and build up to combining different journeys (eg, a train then a bus).
- Be prepared to negotiate. Some group members may need a time limit or ground rules, especially if this is an area of special interest (eg, only one mode of transport allowed, using various routes). Some group members may need a lot of help to negotiate and compromise and to learn to agree or disagree.

Independence levels

Emerging independence

Further activities to develop prerequisite skills include:

- Treasure hunt (Activity 25) can be used to observe the group members' ability to interpret instructions (verbal and/or visual), follow directions and recognise key features in the environment.

Routledge
Taylor & Francis Group

Group members may need support in the following aspects of this activity:

- Making enquiries or bookings, either in person or over the telephone.
- Deciding on the most appropriate mode of transport to use.
- Using maps, plans and timetables.

Facilitating independence

- Group members negotiate roles within the activity (eg, phoning to make enquiries, writing down the questions to ask, recording the information gained, buying tickets or asking for help).

Routledge
Taylor & Francis Group
ROUTLEDGE

G Shopping

Equipment   Funding for the visit (including transport)
Computer
Catalogues or magazines

Top tips

- Be aware of sensory issues (eg, noise, lights, people).
- At both levels, support may be needed to help with negotiation and compromise.
- A high level of support may be needed to help with organisation (eg, locating items in a shop, asking for help, understanding what items a shop sells).
- Be supportive to group members who may display anxieties about being in such an environment.
- If the group have chosen to visit a supermarket to make something for the group to eat, be aware of the layout, where the trolleys are and the position of different checkouts (eg, hand baskets only, 10 items or less). Also consider busy times.
- Be aware of a large group in a small shop/supermarket aisle and the effect this may have on other users. Encourage group members to pair up and find items on a group shopping list and get them to pay for these. Choose pairs carefully.
- The group members all meet at a designated point.
- Provide advice on how to pack goods so none is damaged.
- Encourage group members to be aware of product ranges, brands and prices. For example, some brands may be more expensive than the shop's own brand which may be better for their budget.

Routledge
Taylor & Francis Group

Independence levels

Emerging independence

Group members may need support in the following aspects of this activity:

- Identifying something they would like to shop for as a group (eg, food for a picnic, equipment for school, books, magazines). Thought showers (Activity 33) can be useful for this.
- Researching products and prices: the group could look in catalogues, magazines and on the internet to help with this and use their findings to form a collage, poster or shopping list.
- Some members may need support to pay for their items.

Facilitating independence

- Group members are given a budget and asked to stick to it. A group budget will add the need for negotiation and compromise. For example, one of our groups chose to make a pizza during one of the sessions, which involved deciding on what they wanted on their pizza and going to the local shop to buy the ingredients. The group members were given a budget of £10 and had to plan the activity around this, considering things such as prices and quantity of ingredients, types of ingredients (eg, frozen, fresh) and also how different brands of foods might affect their budget.
- Introduce Public transport (Community visit F) where possible.
- Group members visit a range of shops to encourage generalisation of skills.
- Group members are encouraged to select an item independently, pay and get the receipt.

This page may be photocopied for instructional use only. *Groupwork for Children with ASD Ages 11–16* © A Eggett, K Old, LA Davidson & C Howe 2008

H Swimming/ leisure centre

 Equipment   Funding for the visit (including transport, entrance fee and snacks if required)
Swimming costumes
Towels
Sports kit/equipment

Top tips

- Be aware of sensory issues (eg, noise, touch, movement, lights, proximity to people).
- Be supportive to group members who may display anxieties about being in such an environment.
- Depending on your group members' needs and abilities, this may require a high staffing ratio.
- At both stages, support may be needed to help with negotiation and compromise.
- Support may also be needed with organisation in the changing rooms (eg, with getting dressed).
- Consider times of visits in order to avoid or be prepared for busy periods.
- Organise a designated meeting point for when group members come out of the changing rooms.
- A timetable may be useful to help to plan travel, changing and swimming time, and to allow for long enough in the pool. This can be prepared with the group in the session before and given to them to take home. The group facilitators retain a copy for reference during the practical session.

Independence levels

Emerging independence

Further activities to develop prerequisite skills include:

- An obstacle course (Activity 15) including dressing tasks may be helpful.

Group members may need support in the following aspects of this activity:

- Sensitivity to issues of self-esteem (eg, regarding body shape, fitness levels).

- Any dressing and motor co-ordination issues.

Facilitating independence

- Group members are given a choice of the activities that are available at the leisure centre.
- Group members are given a budget and asked to stick to it. A group budget will add the need for negotiation and compromise.
- Introduce Public transport (Community visit F) where possible.
- Group facilitators should check session times and costs in advance.
- Group members are encouraged to telephone the leisure centre if they think this will be necessary to book an activity (eg, badminton courts).
- Group members are encouraged to pay and get a receipt for their own activity.
- Negotiate which activity would suit most group members or whether they need to split into pairs or smaller groups.

Routledge Taylor & Francis Group   P This page may be photocopied for instructional use only. *Groupwork for Children with ASD Ages 11–16* © A Eggett, K Old, LA Davidson & C Howe 2008

Ⅰ Take-away

Equipment
Telephone

Funding for take-away food

Top tips

- At the emerging independence stage, you may want to demonstrate aspects of this activity to group members (eg, telephoning an order).
- Have a range of menus available (eg, pizza, Chinese, Thai, Indian).
- Consider opening times to fit in with the timing of the group.
- Check the length of the delivery time and that they will deliver to your setting.
- Be aware of the need for negotiation. Some group members may need a time limit and ground rules (eg, only one pizza allowed, which type of take-away). Some group members will need a lot of support to negotiate and compromise.
- Be sensitive to the group member telephoning. Observe for any anxieties. He may need to do this away from the group. A script or notes from a thought shower (Activity 33) may be useful to support them in this.

Independence levels

Emerging independence

Group members may need support in the following aspects of this activity:

- Deciding on the type of food and what to order
- Ordering over the telephone
- Accepting the delivery and paying

Facilitating independence

- Team members negotiate roles within the activity (eg, writing down the orders, placing the orders by telephone, paying for the take-away when it arrives and preparing the tables and drinks).

Routledge
Taylor & Francis Group
ROUTLEDGE

⒥ Team games

Equipment Equipment to play the selected team game (eg, football)
Funding for public transport if appropriate

Top tips

- Group members' previous experiences of team games may have been very negative in the past and may influence their self-esteem and motivation.
- Be aware of group members' needs and sensory issues and adapt activities accordingly (eg, allowing a young person with tactile defensiveness to play in goal will reduce the need for physical proximity to others).
- Many young people with ASD do not tolerate losing; therefore, pay particular attention to praising achievements, discussing feelings evoked by losing and developing coping strategies to manage these situations more effectively.

Independence levels

Emerging independence

- Group members decide on a game to play (eg, football, rounders, cricket).
- A location is selected by the group facilitator (eg, park, leisure centre).
- The group members travel to the venue and carry out the activity.

Further activities to develop prerequisite skills include:

- Activities such as Circuits (Activity 14), Obstacle course (Activity 15), Relays (Activity 16) and Zoo (Activity 23) can be used to develop co-ordination and general movement.
- Role plays (Activity 31), Act out emotions (Activity 34) and Emotional thermometers (Activity 36) can be used to explore the emotions evoked during these activities.

Group members may need support in the following aspects of this activity:

- Picking teams to ensure all group members are included
- Taking turns and understanding rules
- Coping with losing

Routledge
Taylor & Francis Group

Facilitating independence

- Introduce Public transport (Community visit F) where possible.
- The group members select an appropriate location (eg, the local park, leisure centre, beach).
- The group members are responsible for sorting themselves into teams by a fair method (eg, names out of a hat, drawing numbers).
- The group members are responsible for identifying, organising and remembering any equipment.

Routledge
Taylor & Francis Group

K Tenpin bowling

 Equipment Funding for the visit (including transport, entrance fee, shoe hire and snacks if required)

Top tips

- Be aware of any sensory issues that group members may have, as bowling alleys tend to be very noisy and bright.
- One game between six young people is normally enough to fill an hour, including time to change shoes at the beginning and end of the game.
- Remember to pre-book the bowling lanes. Do not forget to specify your groups' needs and ask how they can cater for you (eg, booking an end bowling alley to minimise sensory overload or distractions).

Independence levels

Emerging independence

Further activities to develop prerequisite skills include:

- Circuits (Activity 14), Obstacle course (Activity 15) and Relays (Activity 16) can be used to develop motor skills and give you a chance to observe group members' ability with dressing skills (eg, taking shoes on and off) and potential sensory issues that may relate to a bowling alley (eg, unwillingness to wear hired shoes).
- Knowing your preferences (Activity 11) to identify and be aware of any potential sensory issues linked with this particular type of activity.

Group members may need support in the following aspects of this activity:

- Taking shoes on and off
- Asking for and knowing their correct shoe size
- Selecting the appropriate size and weight of ball
- Holding and throwing the ball
- Turn-taking within the team
- Working as a team to encourage others to reach a common goal
- Using the computer or telling attendants their names for the computer

Groupwork for Children with ASD Ages 11–16 © A Eggett, K Old, LA Davidson & C Howe 2008

Routledge
Taylor & Francis Group
ROUTLEDGE

○ Coping with sensory issues (noise, lighting, movements, proximity to others, tactile issues)

Facilitating independence

○ Encourage group members to pay and consider issues such as budgeting.
○ Introduce Public transport (Community visit F) where possible.

Routledge
Taylor & Francis Group
ROUTLEDGE

Appendices

Appendix I

Group referral form

NAME _____ DATE OF BIRTH _____

ADDRESS _____

PARENT'S/CARER'S NAME _____ TELEPHONE _____

DIAGNOSIS _____

Please give a description of the young person's:

LANGUAGE AND COMMUNICATION SKILLS

SOCIALISATION

LEISURE TIME/INTERESTS

SENSORY ISSUES

MOTOR SKILLS

EMOTIONS/BEHAVIOURAL ISSUES

Routledge
Taylor & Francis Group

NEED TO DEVELOP COPING STRATEGIES/SELF-AWARENESS OF NEEDS

AWARENESS OF DIAGNOSIS

LEVEL OF INDEPENDENCE AND DAILY LIVING SKILLS

IS THE YOUNG PERSON FACING ANY TRANSITIONS IN THE NEXT SIX MONTHS? (eg, moving school)

ARE THERE ANY CONCERNS ABOUT THEIR MENTAL HEALTH?

WHICH PROFESSIONALS ARE INVOLVED WITH THE YOUNG PERSON?

OTHER RELEVANT INFORMATION

PARENT'S/CARER'S CONSENT

REFERRER'S SIGNATURE   **DATE**

REFERRER'S CONTACT DETAILS

Appendix II

Consent form

NAME OF GROUP MEMBER

DATE OF BIRTH

Dear

As part of some group activities we may be video recording and taking photographs to help record your child's progress. We may also go on community visits.

Please sign below to give consent for these activities.

	Signed	Date	Relationship to child
Photographs			
Video			
Community visits			

Please indicate any special dietary requirements and/or allergies your child has (as the children may be offered a snack) and any health/medication issues that we should be aware of:

Yours sincerely

Group facilitator   Date

Routledge
Taylor & Francis Group

Appendix III

Session plan sheet – emerging independence stage

DATE OF SESSION | LOCATION

SESSION START TIME | SESSION END TIME

GROUP FACILITATORS

GENERAL AIMS OF THE SESSION

Warm-up activity	Estimated time
Activity 1	Estimated time
Activity 2	Estimated time
Activity 3	Estimated time
Snack time	Estimated time
Activity 4	Estimated time
Activity 5	Estimated time
Activity 6	Estimated time
Round-up activity	Estimated time

COMMENTS (to be completed after peer review)

RESOURCES NEEDED

SIGNED   DATE

Routledge
Taylor & Francis Group

Appendix IV

Session plan sheet – facilitating independence stage

DATE OF SESSION [   ]   LOCATION [   ]

SESSION START TIME [   ]   SESSION END TIME [   ]

GROUP FACILITATORS [   ]

GENERAL AIMS OF THE SESSION [   ]

Activities	Estimated time

Routledge
Taylor & Francis Group
ROUTLEDGE

Session plan sheet –
facilitating independence stage

COMMENTS (to be completed after peer review)

RESOURCES NEEDED

SIGNED

DATE

Routledge
Taylor & Francis Group
ROUTLEDGE

Appendix V

Group timetable – eight weeks

LOCATION [ ] DATE TIMETABLE COMPLETED [ ]

GROUP FACILITATORS PRESENT [ ]

NAMES OF GROUPWORK PARTICIPANTS [ ]

Session number	Session focus
1	
2	
3	
4	
5	
6	
7	
8	

Routledge
Taylor & Francis Group

ROUTLEDGE

Appendix VI

Group timetable – eighteen weeks

LOCATION [   ]   DATE TIMETABLE COMPLETED [   ]

GROUP FACILITATORS PRESENT [   ]

NAMES OF GROUPWORK PARTICIPANTS [   ]

Session number	Session focus
1	
2	
3	
4	
5	
6	
7	
8	
9	
10	
11	
12	
13	
14	
15	
16	
17	
18	

Routledge
Taylor & Francis Group

Appendix VII

Collage box contents

A good-sized toolbox makes an excellent storage place for collage equipment as it opens out to allow group members to access the things inside and helps to keep the items together in one place, minimising loss of materials.

The following are useful things to consider as contents for a collage box:

Coloured card/paper

Coloured matchsticks

Coloured string

Cotton wool

Crayons

Feathers

Glitter

Glue

Paints/brushes

Paper clips

Pasta

Pencils

Pens

Ruler

Scissors (including left-hand ones)

Split peas

Split pins

Stamps and ink pads

Stencils

Stickers

Things to draw around (eg, cotton reels, paper cups)

Tissue paper

Routledge
Taylor & Francis Group

Appendix VIII

Group summary report

NAME [   ]   DATE OF BIRTH [   ]

DATE GROUP STARTED [   ]   DATE GROUP FINISHED [   ]

NUMBER OF SESSIONS ATTENDED [   ]

GROUP LOCATION [   ]

GROUP FACILITATORS [   ]

AIMS

SUMMARY

RECOMMENDATIONS

SIGNED [*Group facilitators*]   DATE [   ]

SIGNED [*Parent/carer*]   DATE [   ]

Routledge
Taylor & Francis Group
ROUTLEDGE

Appendix IX

Group member evaluation form – emerging independence stage

NAME

DATE

1 Name three things you liked about the group.

2 Name three things you did not like about the group.

3 If you could change something about the group, what would it be?

4 Can you list something you have learned in the group?

5 Would you like to be invited back to another group?

Thank you for coming to our group and giving your opinions. We will use what you have written to make the group better next time.

Routledge
Taylor & Francis Group

Appendix X

Group member evaluation form – facilitating independence stage continued

NAME

DATE

1   Have you enjoyed coming to the group?

Yes ☐   No ☐

2   List three things you have enjoyed about the group.

3   List three things you have not enjoyed about the group.

4   List three things or skills you have learned or developed in the group.

5   Do you feel the venue was appropriate for the group?

Yes ☐   No ☐

Please explain why.

Routledge
Taylor & Francis Group

6 Do you feel that there were enough sessions?

Yes ☐   No ☐

Please explain why.

_____

_____

_____

_____

7 If you were to come to another group, what issues, themes and activities would you like to explore?

Friendships	☐	Going out	☐	Group discussion	☐
Role play/videoing	☐	Diagnosis	☐	Anger	☐
School	☐	Independence	☐	Coping strategies	☐

Can you think of any others?

_____

_____

_____

_____

Thank you for coming to our group and giving your opinions. We will use what you have written to make the group better next time.

Appendix XI

Parent/carer evaluation form (1 of 2)

NAME

PARENT/CARER OF

DATE

1 How convenient was it to attend the group?

Convenient ☐   Not convenient ☐

Comments

2 How suitable was the location of the group?

Suitable ☐   Not suitable ☐

Comments

3 Was the number of sessions:

Too many? ☐   Just right? ☐   Not enough? ☐

Comments

4 Was the length of the sessions:

Too long? ☐   Just right? ☐   Not long enough? ☐

Comments

Routledge
Taylor & Francis Group

5 What were your expectations of the group?

6 Were these expectations met?

7 Do you feel that your son/daughter enjoyed the group?

8 Do you feel that your son/daughter has benefited from the group?

9 Would you bring your son/daughter to another group?

10 If you could change anything about the group, what would it be?

Thank you for taking the time to complete this questionnaire. This helps us to plan future groups.

Routledge
Taylor & Francis Group
ROUTLEDGE

Appendix XII

Session record sheet – emerging independence stage

(1 of 2)

NAME OF GROUP MEMBER		DATE OF BIRTH	
DATE OF SESSION		LOCATION	
SESSION START TIME		SESSION END TIME	
GROUP FACILITATORS			
GROUP MEMBER'S TARGETS			

Warm-up activity
Activity 1
Activity 2
Activity 3
Snack time
Activity 4
Activity 5
Activity 6
Round-up activity

P This page may be photocopied for instructional use only. *Groupwork for Children with ASD Ages 11–16* © A Eggett, K Old, LA Davidson & C Howe 2008

Routledge Taylor & Francis Group

ADDITIONAL COMMENTS (observations relating to mood, activity levels, etc)

AREAS TO BE TARGETED NEXT SESSION

SIGNED *Group facilitator* **DATE**

SIGNED *Group facilitator* **DATE**

Routledge
Taylor & Francis Group

Appendix XIII

Session record sheet –
facilitating independence stage

NAME OF GROUP MEMBER [   ] DATE OF BIRTH [   ]

DATE OF SESSION [   ] LOCATION [   ]

SESSION START TIME [   ] SESSION END TIME [   ]

GROUP FACILITATORS [   ]

GROUP MEMBER'S TARGETS [   ]

ACTIVITIES AND OBSERVATIONS

ADDITIONAL COMMENTS (observations relating to mood, activity levels, etc)

AREAS TO BE TARGETED NEXT SESSION

SIGNED [*Group facilitator*] DATE [   ]

SIGNED [*Group facilitator*] DATE [   ]

Routledge
Taylor & Francis Group
ROUTLEDGE

Appendix XIV

People bingo

NAME

Loves music	Is left-handed
Can roll their tongue	Hates loud noises
Has dark hair	Is wearing something black

Routledge
Taylor & Francis Group
ROUTLEDGE

Appendix XV

People bingo – blank

NAME

Appendix XVI

Interview sheet

NAME OF INTERVIEWEE

NAME OF INTERVIEWER

DATE

1 Where do you go to school?

2 Which teacher is your least favourite and why?

3 Do you prefer dogs or cats?

4 Have you got any talents and skills, or is there anything you are good at?

5 What makes you happy?

Routledge
Taylor & Francis Group
ROUTLEDGE

Appendix XVII

Interview sheet – blank

NAME OF INTERVIEWEE

NAME OF INTERVIEWER

DATE

1 Question

Answer

2 Question

Answer

3 Question

Answer

Routledge
Taylor & Francis Group
ROUTLEDGE

Appendix XVIII

Show and tell letter to home

Date _____

Dear _____ (group member)

For the next session, please bring something that is very special to you. We would like you to show it to the rest of the group. Good things to bring would be a favourite book, item of sports equipment or a game.

If it is valuable, breakable or alive, please do not bring it to the group. Instead you could bring in a photograph of it.

Thank you

_____

Group facilitators

Routledge
Taylor & Francis Group
ROUTLEDGE

Appendix XIX

Activities card template

You can use the template below to make your own cards for Hangman (Activity 12), Charades (Activity 20), Say the picture (Activity 21) and Act out emotions (Activity 34).

Appendix XX

Sensory box contents

The following is a list of ideas for equipment and objects to include in a sensory box. See the List of suppliers (Appendix XXV) for further details.

Bells

Bouncing balls

Bubble wrap

Bubbles

Cotton wool

Cymbals

Elastic balls

Feathers

Flashing toys

Glitter tubes

Goo in a pot

Hologram paper or disks

Jelly-filled balls

Jelly toys

Laser lights

Lava lamps

Oil tubes

Pin art

Pine cones

Playdough

Rain stick

Rattles

Scrubbing brush

Shaving foam

Silk fabric

Spinning tops

Spinning toys with lights

Squashy balls with objects inside (eg, plastic worms)

Sound tubes

Triangle

Velvet fabric

Vibrating toys and animals

Whistles

Appendix XXI

ASD quiz questions

These questions should be used with careful consideration to the group members. Only ask them if it is relevant to their targets, level of awareness, insight and acceptance of their diagnosis of ASD.

- ○ True or false: more boys than girls have ASD.

- ○ True or false: people with ASD are not as intelligent as other people.

- ○ True or false: ASD is more common in English-speaking countries.

- ○ What are the three main areas that people with ASD have difficulty with?

- ○ What do the letters ASD stand for?

- ○ How long has ASD been known about?

- ○ Other than in the three main areas of social skills, communication and imagination, what other difficulties can people with ASD have?

- ○ True or false: all boys with ASD love trains.

- ○ Name one famous person who has characteristics of ASD.

- ○ Why do some people with ASD not like eating certain foods?

- ○ Do individuals with ASD show affection?

- ○ True or false: all people with ASD have problems with friendships.

- ○ Can you think of positive attributes of ASD?

Routledge
Taylor & Francis Group

Appendix XXII

The brain

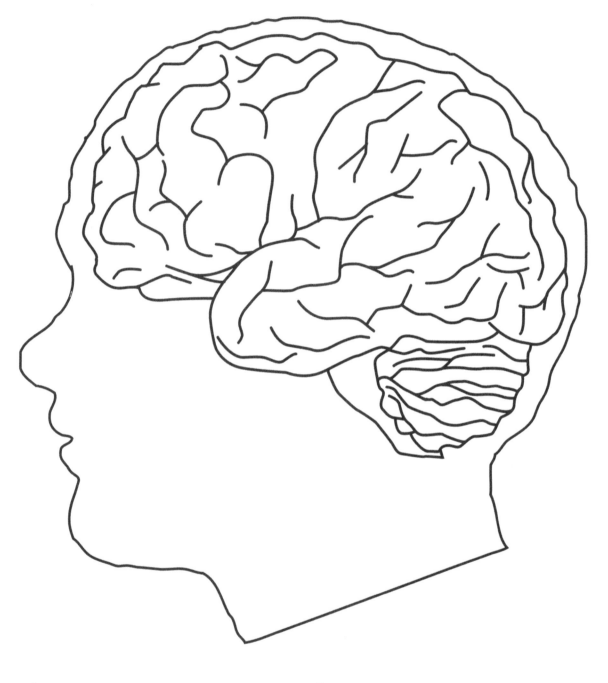

1 ....   6 ....

2 ....   7 ....

3 ....   8 ....

4 ....   9 ....

5 ....   10 ....

Routledge
Taylor & Francis Group
ROUTLEDGE

Appendix XXIII

Emotional thermometer

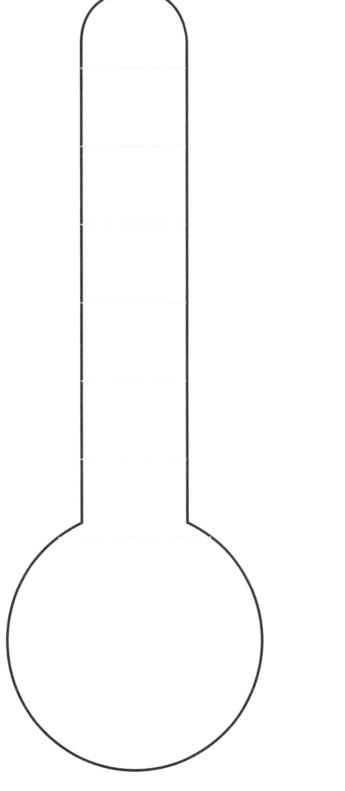

The feeling we are describing is _____

Routledge
Taylor & Francis Group

Ideas for circuits, obstacle courses and relays

All of the activities below can be used for a circuit, obstacle course or relay. The number of activities you choose depends on the ability of the group and level of the activity you are working to.

We are aware that some of the activities below require specialist equipment (see Appendix XXV for a List of suppliers). We have, therefore, divided the activities into ones that need equipment and those that do not. This means you will still be able to carry out a circuit, obstacle course or relay even if you have no equipment available.

Activities that do not need equipment

Bunny hops

○ Crouch down with your hands and feet on the floor. With your knees between your elbows, jump forwards to return to your original position.

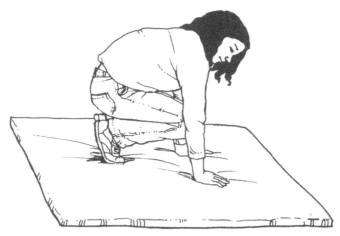

Jump forwards

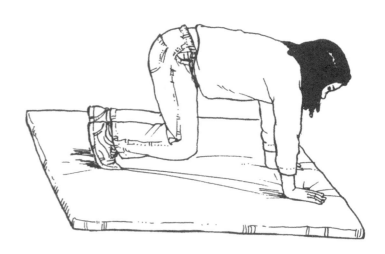

Start and finish position

Routledge
Taylor & Francis Group

Crab walking

○ With your feet on the floor, lie backwards, supported by your hands (the front of your body should be facing up towards the ceiling). Holding this position, move sideways.

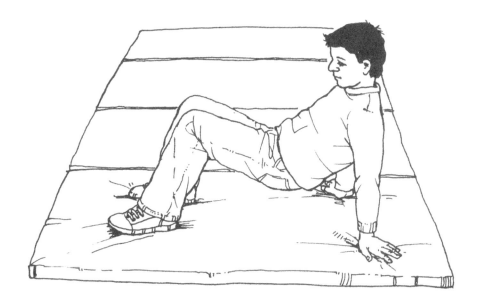

Hopping

○ Standing on one leg, hop up and down on the spot or move forwards/backwards.

Jumping

○ Standing with feet together, jump up and down on the spot or move forwards/backwards.

Rolling

○ Lie on your back with your arms stretched out above your head. Roll to the side.

Running on the spot

○ Run in one place (without moving forwards/backwards).

Stretching

○ Hold a number of different stretches (eg, stand with arms above head, stand with one arm stretched across the body, stretch one leg out behind you when standing).

Routledge
Taylor & Francis Group

Star jumps

○ Stand with feet together and arms by your sides. Jump your feet apart sideways at the same time as raising your arms from your sides so they are parallel to the floor. Jump back into your original position.

Wheelbarrows

○ This needs two people. One person lies on their front on the floor. The other person stands at their feet. The standing person lifts the other person's feet off the floor. The person lying on the floor raises themselves onto their hands so their body is off the ground. The pair then walk forwards, holding this position.

Activities needing equipment

Ball games

○ Bounce the ball on the ground and catch it. Choose the number of repetitions according to the ability of group members. At the basic level, bounce the ball on the spot. To make it more difficult, and if room allows, you may move with the ball.

○ Throw the ball in the air and catch it. Vary how many times you do this according to the ability of the group members. At the basic level, catch the ball on the spot. To make it more difficult, and if room allows, you may move with the ball.

○ Throw the ball at a target. Repeat according to the ability of the group members. This is a static activity that does not allow for moving about; however, if a group member is finding it too easy you may move them further from the target. Likewise, if it is too difficult, move them closer to it.

Beanbags

○ These are useful bits of 'treasure' to be collected while group members are on the scooter board, wobble board or stepping stones. They can also be collected by teams during relays.

Beanbags and hoop

○ Throw a beanbag into a hoop. Alter the number of bags that need to be thrown into the hoop according to the ability of the group member.

○ Increase the distance from the hoop.

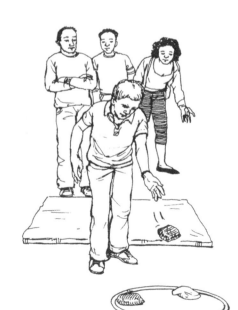

Routledge
Taylor & Francis Group
ROUTLEDGE

Bench

- Walk along the bench holding the group facilitator's hand.
- Walk along independently.
- Step up and step down from the bench.

Cones

- These are placed in a line. More or less cones can be added according to the ability of group members.
- Walk in and out of the cones.
- Wheelbarrow in and out of them.
- Dribble a ball around the cones.
- Crab walk around the cones.
- Hop around the cones.

Dart board and darts (eg, magnetic)

- Start near the board and move further away as the group member becomes more skilled.

Dressing-up box

- This can be used in the relay or obstacle course. Each person needs to collect a piece of clothing as they go and place it on another group member during a relay or on a group facilitator at the end of an obstacle course.
- It can be an activity in itself for circuits (eg, stand on the spot and put on five different pieces of clothing).

Mats

- Use for rolling or for providing a soft landing for activities such as the mini-trampoline and wobble board.
- Mats can be used as a marker for the beginning/end of the obstacle course, circuit or relay.

Mini-trampoline

- This can be used for jumping up and down.
- To make it more difficult, this can be done while clapping or catching a ball.

Routledge
Taylor & Francis Group

Scooter board

Group members should lie flat on their front with their stomach on the board, manoeuvring around obstacles.

Scooter board and rope

This activity requires more than one person.

One group member sits or lies on the scooter board. They pull themselves along on a rope held up by two people.

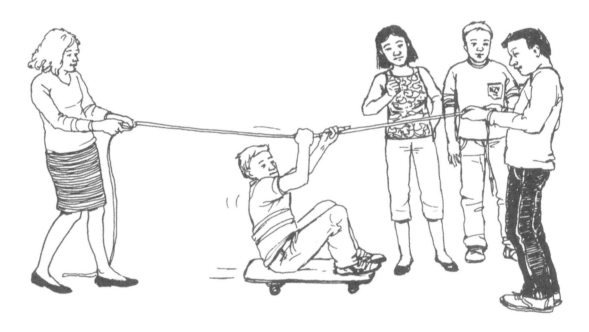

Skipping rope

Group members could skip forwards and backwards on the spot as part of your obstacle course or circuit, or have a skipping race within a relay.

Stepping stones

Alter the number of stepping stones used, and the distance placed between them, depending on the individual group member's motor planning skills (eg, a group member with poor balance may need fewer stepping stones placed closer together).

Therapy ball

- The ball should remain in the same spot whilst the group member is bouncing up and down in a sitting position.
- Group members lie face down with their stomach on the stationary ball, trying to collect objects from the floor (eg, beanbags).

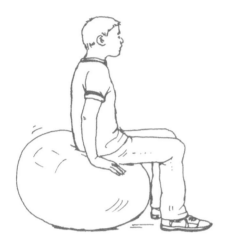 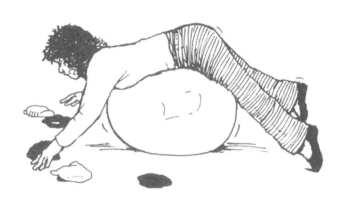

Tunnel

- Group members move from one end of the tunnel through to the other.
- Place beanbags or other objects in the tunnel for group members to collect (eg, clothing – see 'Dressing-up box' above).

Wobble board

- This often needs one-to-one supervision as group members with poor balance may fall off.
- Wobble boards are designed so that you stand with feet on either side and wobble to move the board. This moves a ball in the centre of the board into a hole.
- Group members stand on the board and move the ball to the centre.

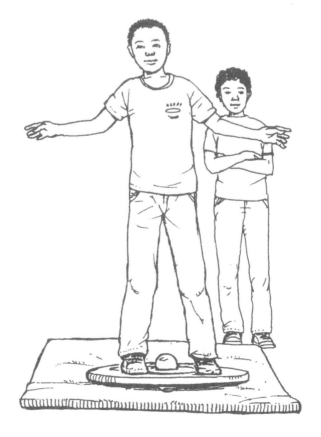

Groupwork for Children with ASD Ages 11–16 © A Eggett, K Old, LA Davidson & C Howe 2008

Routledge
Taylor & Francis Group
ROUTLEDGE

Appendix XXV

List of suppliers

Acorn Educational
27 The Woodlands
Geddington
Kettering
Northants
NN14 1BE

Tel 01536 747485
sales@acorneducational.co.uk

Innovations
Davies Sports
Lee Fold
Hyde
Cheshire
SK14 4LL

Tel 0845 1204515
enquiries@daviessports.co.uk

James Galt and Co Ltd
Sovereign House
Stockport Road
Cheadle
Cheshire
SK8 2EA

Tel 0161 4289111
www.galt.co.uk

Nottingham Rehab
Findel House
Excelsior Road
Ashby De La Zouch
Leicestershire
LE65 1NG

Tel 0845 1204522
www.nrs-uk.co.uk

ROMPA
Goyt Side Road
Chesterfield
Derbyshire
S40 2PH

Tel 01246 211777
www.rompa.com

SpaceKraft Ltd
Titus House
29 Saltaire Road
Shipley
West Yorks
BD18 3HH

Tel 01274 581007
www.spacekraft.co.uk

Special Direct @TTS
Park Lane Business Park
Kirby-In-Ashfield
Nottinghamshire
NG17 9LE

Tel 0800 318686
sales@tts-group.co.uk

Appendix XXVI

Anger wordsearch

Find these words in the grid. They may be in any direction: forwards, backwards or diagonally.

breathing   calm   control   cross

face   help   mad   rage

thoughts   violent

g	r	e	e	t	k	r	x	g	e	f	k	v	f	d
e	z	q	i	o	j	b	n	h	g	w	w	o	k	g
y	b	w	c	a	y	i	c	d	a	z	d	v	n	f
x	a	h	x	a	h	h	o	w	r	d	h	i	u	u
m	l	a	c	t	h	o	u	g	h	t	s	o	p	z
h	j	k	a	c	i	c	m	a	d	q	x	l	t	z
x	m	e	h	x	r	v	e	b	q	w	e	e	e	n
a	r	u	p	o	y	z	n	c	v	h	f	n	r	d
b	a	u	s	c	l	g	n	z	a	m	y	t	n	y
u	m	s	m	o	o	s	r	h	c	f	e	h	c	k
n	q	z	d	q	u	n	g	i	d	n	x	h	u	w
z	t	m	w	u	y	c	t	m	v	m	u	t	g	y
o	g	m	c	y	z	d	d	r	c	z	d	j	z	v
d	x	a	z	c	w	s	m	h	o	q	s	w	h	l
c	l	m	g	x	t	q	s	v	f	l	w	q	i	a

Recommended reading

Attwood T, 1997, *Asperger's Syndrome: A Guide for Parents and Professionals*, Jessica Kingsley Publishers, London.

Bogdashina O, 2003, *Sensory Perceptual Issues in Autism and Asperger Syndrome: Different Sensory Experiences, Different Perceptual Worlds*, Jessica Kingsley Publishers, London.

Bogdashina O, 2005, *Communication Issues in Autism and Asperger Syndrome: Do We Speak the Same Language?*, Jessica Kingsley Publishers, London.

Ghaziuddin M, 2005, *Mental Health Aspects of Autism and Asperger Syndrome*, Jessica Kingsley Publishers, London.

Gutstein SE & Sheely RK, 2002, *Relationship Development Intervention with Children, Adolescents and Adults*, Jessica Kingsley Publishers, London.

Holliday Willey L (ed), 2003, *Asperger Syndrome in Adolescence: Living with the Ups, the Downs and Things in Between*, Jessica Kingsley Publishers, London.

Howlin P, Baron-Cohen S & Hadwin J, 1998, *Teaching Children with Autism to Mind-Read: A Practical Guide*, Wiley, Chichester.

Leicester City Council and Leicestershire County Council, 1998, *Asperger Syndrome – Practical Strategies for the Classroom: A Teacher's Guide*, National Autistic Society, London.

Lougher L, 2000, *Occupational Therapy for Child and Adolescent Mental Health*, Churchill Livingstone/Harcourt Publishers, London.

Miller-Kuhaneck H, 2004, *Autism: A Comprehensive Occupational Therapy Approach*, 2nd edn, American Occupational Therapy Association, Maryland, MD.

Murray D (ed), 2005, *Coming Out Asperger: Diagnosis, Disclosure and Self-Confidence*, Jessica Kingsley Publishers, London.

Murray-Slutsky C & Paris BA, 2000, *Exploring the Spectrum of Autism and Pervasive Developmental Disorder Intervention Strategies*, Therapy Skill Builders, San Antonio, TX.

Northumberland County Council Communication Support Services, 2005, *Autism Spectrum Disorders: Practical Strategies for Teachers and Other Professionals*, David Fulton Publishers Ltd, London.

Smith Myles B, Tapscott Cook K, Miller NE, Rinner L & Robbins LA, 2001, *Asperger Syndrome and Sensory Issues: Practical Solutions for Making Sense of the World*, Jessica Kingsley Publishers, London.

Stuart L, Wright F, Grigor S & Howey A, 2002, *Spoken Language Difficulties: Practical Strategies and Activities for Teachers and Other Professionals*, David Fulton Publishers Ltd, London.

Thomas R & Whitman L, 2004, *The Development of Autism: A Self-Regulatory Perspective*, Jessica Kingsley Publishers, London.

Welton J, 2003, *Can I Tell You About Asperger Syndrome? A Guide for Friends and Family*, Jessica Kingsley Publishers, London.

Personal accounts of ASD

Hoopmann K, 2003, *Haze*, Jessica Kingsley Publishers, London.

Jackson L, 2002, *Freaks, Geeks & Asperger Syndrome: A User Guide to Adolescence*, Jessica Kingsley Publishers, London.

Sainsbury C, 2000, *Martian in the Playground: Understanding the Schoolchild with Asperger's Syndrome*, Lucky Duck Publishing Ltd, Bristol.

References

Aarons M & Gittens T, 1992, *The Handbook of Autism: A Guide for Parents and Professionals*, Routledge, London.

American Psychiatric Association, 1994, *Diagnostic and Statistical Manual IV*, APA, Washington, DC.

Bundy AC, Lane SJ & Murray EA, 2002, *Sensory Integration Theory and Practice*, 2nd edn, FA Davis Company, Philadelphia, PA.

Clegg J, Hollis C & Rutter Sir M, 1999, 'Life sentence: What Happens to Children with Developmental Language Disorders in Later Life?', *RCSLT Bulletin November*, pp16–18.

Crossley D, 2000, *Muddles, Puddles and Sunshine*, Hawthorn Press, Stroud.

DfES, 2003, *Every Child Matters: Summary of Green Paper*, Department for Education and Skills, HMSO. © Crown Copyright 1995–2003.

Dunn W, 1999, *The Sensory Profile*, The Psychological Corporation, TX.

Frith U (ed), 1991, *Autism and Asperger Syndrome*, Cambridge University Press, Cambridge.

Howe C, Old K, Eggett A & Davidson LA, 2008, *Groupwork for Children with Autism Spectrum Disorder Ages 5–11: An Integrated Approach*, Speechmark Publishing, Milton Keynes.

Kashman N & Mora J, 2002, *The Sensory Connection: An OT and SLP Team Approach*, Sensory Resources LLC, Las Vegas, NV.

Sparrow SS, 1984, *Vineland Adaptive Behavior Scales*, AGS, Minnesota, MN.

Sunderland M & Engleheart P, 1993, *Draw on Your Emotions: Creative Ways to Explore, Express and Understand Important Feelings*, Speechmark Publishing, Milton Keynes.

Watson D, Townsley R, Abbott D & Latham P, 2002, *Working Together? Multi-Agency Working in Services to Disabled Children with Complex Needs and their Families: A Literature Review*, Handsel Trust Publications, Birmingham.

Wing L, 1995, *Autistic Spectrum Disorders: An Aid to Diagnosis*, National Autistic Society, London.

World Health Organisation, 1993, *The ICD-10 Classification of Mental and Behavioural Disorders: Diagnostic Criteria for Research*, WHO, Geneva.

Wright JA & Kersner M, 1998, *Supporting Children with Communication Problems: Sharing the Workload*, David Fulton Publishers Ltd, London.

*For Product Safety Concerns and Information please contact
our EU representative GPSR@taylorandfrancis.com Taylor & Francis
Verlag GmbH, Kaufingerstraße 24, 80331 München, Germany*

T - #0002 - 160425 - C0 - 297/210/14 - SB - 9780863885952 - Gloss Lamination